PROMOTING CHILDREN'S HEALTH

Promoting Children's Health

Integrating School, Family, and Community

THOMAS J. POWER
GEORGE J. DuPAUL
EDWARD S. SHAPIRO
ANNE E. KAZAK

THE GUILFORD PRESS
New York   London

To our families
  Whose love nourishes our work,
To the children and families we serve
  Who challenge us to keep our work real,
And to our mentors, colleagues, and students
  Who encourage us to question paradigms
  to promote the health of all children.

Library of Congress Cataloging-in-Publication Data

Promoting children's health : integrating school, family, and community
/ Thomas J. Power . . . [et al.].
       p. cm.
Includes bibliographical references and index.
   ISBN 1-57230-855-9 (alk. paper)
   1. Children—Health and hygiene. 2. Child mental health services. 3.
School health services. I. Power, Thomas J.
RJ101.P686 2003
                                                      2002151193

About the Authors

Thomas J. Power, PhD, Associate Professor of School Psychology in Pediatrics at the University of Pennsylvania School of Medicine, is Program Director of the Center for Management of ADHD and Community Schools Program at the Children's Hospital of Philadelphia. A Fellow of the American Psychological Association (APA, Division 16), he is Associate Editor of *School Psychology Review* and has coauthored numerous journal articles as well as several books, including *Pediatric Psychopharmacology: Combining Medical and Psychosocial Interventions* (APA) and *Homework Success for Children with ADHD: A Family–School Intervention Program* (Guilford Press). Dr. Power is Co-Director (with Drs. Shapiro and DuPaul) of a training project funded by the U.S. Department of Education to prepare school psychologists to integrate systems of care to promote children's health and prevent mental health disorders.

George J. DuPaul, PhD, is Professor and Coordinator of School Psychology at Lehigh University, Bethlehem, Pennsylvania. His primary research interests are the school-based treatment of disruptive behavior disorders as well as school-based interventions for children with chronic health conditions. He is the author of over 100 journal articles and book chapters regarding the assessment and treatment of attention-deficit/hyperactivity disorder. His other books include *ADHD in the Schools: Assessment and Intervention Strategies* (second edition) and *ADHD Rating Scale–IV: Checklists, Norms, and Clinical Interpretation*, both published by The Guilford Press. Dr. DuPaul has served as an Associate Editor for *School Psychology Review* and *School Psychology Quarterly*. He is a Fellow of Divisions 16 (School Psychology) and 53 (Clinical Child Psychology) of the American Psychological Association.

Edward S. Shapiro, PhD, Iacocca Professor of Education, Professor of School Psychology, and Chairperson of the Department of Education and Human Services at Lehigh University, Bethlehem, Pennsylvania, is the author or coauthor of several books, including his most recent edited volumes, *Conducting School-Based Assessments of Child and Adolescent Behavior* and *Behavioral Assessment in Schools: Theory, Research, and Clinical Implications* (second edition), both published by The Guilford Press. Recipient of over $7 million in research and training grants, he is co-directing a federal training project focused on developing doctoral school psychologists as pediatric school psychologists (a model for training students to integrate the health, psychological, and educational needs of children within school settings), as well as a project focused on training school psychologists to be effective interventionists for the inclusion of students with low-incidence disabilities into general education settings.

Anne E. Kazak, PhD, ABPP, is Director of the Department of Psychology at the Children's Hospital of Philadelphia and Professor and Director of Psychology Research in the Department of Pediatrics at the University of Pennsylvania. Dr. Kazak received her PhD in Clinical–Community Psychology in 1983 from the University of Virginia and completed her internship training at Yale University School of Medicine, Department of Psychiatry. She is the incoming Editor of the *Journal of Family Psychology* and the immediate past Editor of the *Journal of Pediatric Psychology*, the official scientific publication of the Society of Pediatric Psychology, Division 54 of the American Psychological Association. Dr. Kazak's research focuses on interventions to enhance adaptive functioning and reduce child and family distress associated with serious pediatric illnesses.

Preface

This book is intended to provide a framework for conceptualizing the roles that healthcare, mental healthcare, and educational professionals can serve in addressing the health needs of children. In this volume, we emphasize both a service delivery approach (i.e., designing interventions for one or more children who have identified concerns) and a public health approach (i.e., creating programs that address the developmental needs of a large group of healthy children or those at risk for problems).

This book should serve as a useful guide for professionals from a wide range of disciplines who address the healthcare and mental healthcare needs of children and their families. A major premise of the book is that professionals must work to integrate systems of care to manage successfully and prevent healthcare concerns (see Chapters 1 and 2). Thus, professionals focusing on a wide range of systems, including the healthcare, school, family, and community systems, will find this text helpful. However, there is a particular focus on addressing the professional issues of psychologists who work with children, including clinical child psychologists, pediatric psychologists, school psychologists, family psychologists, and community psychologists.

Practitioners will find this text useful, because it offers models and provides specific guidelines for developing and evaluating programs of intervention and prevention. Also, case examples are included to illustrate methods for applying evidence-based strategies in practice. In this volume, topics related to intervention include (1) integrating assessment paradigms to design successful intervention strategies, (2) developing strategies to promote the successful integration of children with health problems into school, (3) forming partnerships to promote intervention adherence, and (4) incorporating pharmacological interventions into the management of health problems (see Chapters 3 through 6). Topics in this text related to prevention include (1) developing selective and indicated prevention programs, (2) developing universal prevention programs, and (3) evaluating programs of prevention (see Chapters 7 through 9).

University trainers at the graduate and undergraduate levels will find this book helpful in preparing students for careers related to the management and prevention of healthcare concerns. Chapter 10, in particular, is useful to trainers in that it provides guidelines for designing programs to prepare professionals for health-related careers. Two model training initiatives, one embedded in a school psychology program and the other in a clinical child psychology program, are described. Finally, researchers and policymakers will appreciate the focus on methods for linking science with practice and for disseminating evidence-based practices, particularly in the final chapter (Chapter 11).

Contents

PART I

Understanding the Context

CHAPTER 1

Linking Systems of Care to Promote Health

Justification and Need

Children with health problems present significant challenges to families, healthcare providers, schools, and communities. Consider the following situation:

> Sherri, 10 years of age, was brought to the emergency department of a nearby hospital after being involved in a car accident. Her father was driving her to a soccer game when the accident occurred. Sherri sustained a brain injury that was considered moderate in severity, as well as a broken right wrist. She was admitted to the hospital for 4 days and then discharged back into the community.

Sherri's medical condition has effects that reverberate throughout the community. Her primary care provider must become involved and assist in the coordination of her medical care and rehabilitation. The school faces the challenge of educating Sherri when her functioning is compromised by both an injury to her writing hand and impairments in attention and memory caused by the head injury. Her family must cope with the short- and long-term effects of the injury on her functioning, as well as her emotional reactions and perhaps the father's guilt.

Sherri's situation, like that of most children with a health condition, presents a real challenge to the community. Reforms in the healthcare system have been spawned in large measure to respond to the complex systems and fiscal issues raised by individuals with conditions such as Sherri's. Health reforms, including the managed care movement, have emphasized that the integration of systems of care is critical to the delivery of quality healthcare services. Furthermore, health reforms have highlighted the importance of developing a comprehensive approach to service delivery that balances a focus on intervention for individual children with or at risk for health problems, with a focus on prevention for groups of children who are healthy and developing appropriately (Knoff, 1996; Short & Talley, 1997).

Changes in social policy, as well as advancements in research, have created the need for professionals who can effectively link systems of care to manage and prevent health problems. The purpose of this chapter is to (1) discuss the reform movements occurring in the fields of health, mental health, and education, and describe their impact on service delivery for children and families; (2) describe some of the major advancements in medicine, psychology, and education that have had led to changes in research and practice; (3) discuss the emerging opportunities and challenges for child-oriented psychologists; and (4) describe the need to link specialties of child psychology with other disciplines to respond to policy reforms and advancements in research related to healthcare.

SOCIOPOLITICAL REFORMS

Reforms occurring in the healthcare, mental healthcare, and educational systems of the United States since the mid-1980s have had a profound impact on the delivery of services for children and families. Although each of these reform movements has developed in response to a different set of pressures and contingencies, they have had a similar impact on service delivery by emphasizing the need for multisystemic integration and the importance of prevention as well as intervention.

Reforms in Healthcare

Chronic health problems, including mental health disorders, among children and adolescents are highly prevalent. The estimated prevalence of one or more mental health disorders among children and adolescents between the ages of 9 and 17 years is 21% (Shaffer et al., 1996), and the prevalence of common health conditions such as obesity and asthma is estimated to be 22% and 10%, respectively (Creer & Bender, 1995; Troiano, Flegal, Kuczmarski, Campbell, & Johnson, 1995). The costs of chronic health conditions, including outpatient and inpatient medical care, residential treatment or placement in the juvenile justice system, and, in some cases, premature death, can be extremely costly to families and to society.

The healthcare reform movement was initiated in response to serious concerns about the rising costs of healthcare and the increasing mortality associated with certain health conditions, in particular, HIV infection and AIDS. A major thrust of the healthcare reform movement has been to shift the focus of healthcare from secondary and tertiary care settings to primary care sites (Dryfoos, 1994). Primary care providers in both the healthcare and mental healthcare sectors have been established as gatekeepers into the system. In many cases, incentives are given to primary care providers to maintain children in community settings and to prevent the delivery of services in more expensive, secondary and tertiary care sites. In the event that hospitalization is indicated, length of stays have been shortened considerably (Roberts & Hurley, 1997). Increasingly, children and their families must rely on systems of support in the community during the period of recovery and rehabilitation. This shift has supported the establishment of full-service schools or community schools in an effort to increase access and provide coordinated care to children and families in the community (Dryfoos, 1994; Reeder et al., 1997).

The service delivery model for children with traumatic brain injury (TBI) serves as an illustration of the shift to a community-based model of care. Historically, the care of children with a moderate to severe TBI often involved a process of acute and rehabilitative care lasting several months. At present, the hospitalization of these children may last only several days, resulting in reentry into the community when the child is still in the relatively early stages of recovery (Farmer, Clippard, Luehr-Wiemann, Wright, & Owings, 1997). The impact of this change has been to increase the responsibility of the healthcare, mental healthcare, school, and family systems to provide rehabilitation to children with TBI and to assist them in their transition back to mainstream settings. Because the care of children and families may involve multiple systems, there has been increased emphasis on the importance of integrating systems and coordinating providers of care (Talley & Short, 1995).

The health reform movement has placed significant emphasis on the prevention of health risk and the promotion of health for all children (Short & Talley, 1997). The focus on prevention has further affirmed the preeminence of community-based models of care. The school, in particular, has been the target of prevention efforts, because it serves the needs of almost all children in the community and has existing mechanisms for coordinating interdisciplinary services for children and families (Kolbe, Collins, & Cortese, 1997). Eight components of school-based health promotion programming have been delineated by the U.S. Public Health Service, Centers for Disease Control, and Division of Adolescent and School Health of the U.S. Department of Health and Human Services.

These include health education for students, physical education, health-care services, nutrition services, health promotion for school staff, coun-seling and social services for children and families, promotion of a healthy school environment, and promotion of community and family involvement (see Talley & Short, 1995).

Developing successful school-based prevention programs requires collaboration among a wide range of potential stakeholders (Dowrick et al., 2001). For example, a highly innovative, school-based obesity pre-vention program has been developed for Native American children through the collaborative efforts of teachers and school administrators, food service personnel, children and their caregivers, and health profes-sionals and researchers from several universities (Gittelsohn et al., 1999). Similarly, effective violence prevention programming in schools typically involves experts from the mental healthcare system, in addition to other relevant stakeholders, including teachers, school administrators, guidance counselors, playground supervisors, children, caregivers, and community leaders (Leff, Power, Manz, Costigan, & Nabors, 2001).

Reforms in Mental Healthcare

Mental health disorders are highly prevalent, but less than 50% of chil-dren and adolescents with these disorders receive services to address their needs from mental health specialists or primary pediatric care pro-viders (U.S. Department of Health and Human Services, 1999). Barriers to care are multifaceted and may include (1) the stigma associated with mental healthcare services; (2) financial costs; (3) transportation, sched-uling, and child care concerns; (4) cultural and familial patterns of help-seeking behavior; (5) family communication patterns; and (6) family dis-satisfaction with services (Bickman & Rog, 1995; Kazdin, Holland, & Crowley, 1997; Logan & King, 2001; Pavuluri, Luk, & McGee, 1996). Barriers to the provision of mental healthcare services have been found to be substantially greater for families from low-income backgrounds, particularly those of ethnic minority status, compared to families with greater socioeconomic resources and those of ethnic majority back-ground (U.S. Department of Health and Human Services, 2001).

The Surgeon General Report on Mental Health (U.S. Department of Health and Human Services, 1999, 2001) has outlined several priorities for mental healthcare reform (see Table 1.1 for a description of these pri-orities and strategies proposed to address each area). A principal area of focus is the destigmatization of mental healthcare. Efforts to reduce stigma need to focus on improving public awareness of the inseparable link between biological and psychosocial factors in contributing to men-tal health problems (U.S. Department of Health and Human Services, 1999). Also, partnership-based models of care involving nonhierarchical

TABLE 1.1. Reform Priorities Outlined in the Surgeon General Report on Mental Health and Proposed Strategies for Addressing Each Priority

Reform priorities	Proposed strategies
1. Build the scientific database.	Conduct studies comparing pharmacological and multicomponent psychosocial treatments.
	Conduct prevention research.
2. Overcome stigma.	Educate public about the biological and psychosocial factors contributing to mental health disorders.
	Develop programs in partnership with community stakeholders.
3. Improve public awareness of effective treatments.	Disseminate information about empirically supported interventions.
	Identify multiple sources of mental health assistance in community.
4. Ensure supply of mental health services.	Enlist and empower natural helpers from the community.
	Coordinate systems of care.
5. Ensure the delivery of state-of-the-art treatments.	Enlist community providers in developing strategies to improve implementation and quality control.
	Bridge the gap between research and practice.
6. Tailor treatment to age, gender, race, and culture.	Use assessment tools that account for age, gender, race, and culture.
	Develop programs in partnership with community stakeholders representing the full range of ages and cultures served.
7. Facilitate entry into treatment.	Understand and be responsive to help-seeking patterns in the community.
	Provide services in multiple settings, including health settings, school, and faith-based centers.
8. Reduce financial barriers to care.	Advocate for legislation that provides equitable insurance coverage for physical and mental healthcare services.
	Reduce the number of children and families who are un- or underinsured.

Note. Priorities and proposed strategies are derived from the U.S. Department of Health and Human Services (1999) and discussed further in Power, Manz, and Leff (in press).

collaboration between mental health specialists and community stakeholders (i.e., school personnel, caregivers, community residents and leaders) during every stage of program development, implementation, and evaluation can improve the social validity of services and reduce stigma (Fantuzzo & Mohr, 2000; Nastasi et al., 2000; Power, Manz, & Leff, in press).

cultural focus

Another priority highlighted in the Surgeon General Report is to facilitate entry into mental healthcare programs. A key strategy in improving entry into services is to understand how families from varying cultures conceptualize children's behavior, make decisions about the need for help, and identify individuals whom they believe can be helpful (McMiller & Weisz, 1996; Pavuluri et al., 1996). It is critical that services be developed in a manner that is responsive to the goals and preferences of families from the diverse cultural backgrounds represented in the community (Dowrick et al., 2001). Fiscal barriers, such as differential reimbursement from third-party payers for physical versus mental healthcare services, also need to be reduced (U.S. Department of Health and Human Services, 1999).

Reforms in Education

Education reforms have emphasized that the mission of schools is to improve instructional outcomes by (1) heightening expectations for student performance and enhancing the quality of instruction, (2) creating rigorous systems of accountability for students and teachers, and (3) addressing potential barriers to instruction (Adelman & Taylor, 1998). Barriers to instruction include a wide range of noninstructional factors, such as the health and mental health of the child, that can have an impact on learning and academic performance (Adelman, 1996). A major act of legislation outlining the framework for educational reform, the Goals 2000: Educate America Act of 1994, highlighted the critical need to create a safe and drug-free school environment for all children. Goals 2000 affirmed that addressing the healthcare needs of children is the business of schools, and that schools have a critical role to serve in providing healthcare services related to intervention and prevention (Short & Talley, 1997; Tharinger et al., 1996).

Reforms in the special education system also have had a significant effect on the delivery of healthcare services to schools. Special education rights have been extended to children with chronic health conditions that can have a significant effect on educational performance (e.g., TBI, attention-deficit/hyperactivity disorder [ADHD], and sickle-cell disease), in addition to persons with traditionally recognized disabilities (e.g., learning disabilities, mental retardation, and emotional disturbance). Special education regulations enacted since the late 1980s (see Individuals with Disabilities Education Act, 1997) have asserted that children with disabilities, even those with severe impairments, generally are entitled to an education in the neighborhood school in classrooms serving primarily healthy children developing within age expectancies.

These educational reforms have shifted the care of children with

special health needs from specialized settings to mainstream school environments. The impact of this change is that school professionals, in
collaboration with the family, are required to provide an appropriate
education for each child in an inclusionary setting. This shift in responsibility has created the need for partnerships between educational, healthcare, and mental healthcare professionals in the delivery of school
services (Adelman & Taylor, 1998).

ADVANCEMENTS IN MEDICINE, PSYCHOLOGY, AND EDUCATION

As reforms in major sociopolitical systems have been unfolding, significant advancements in research and practice have occurred in the fields of
medicine and psychology. These developments have reinforced the importance of linking systems of care in the community to manage and
prevent health problems and to promote healthy behavior.

Rapid Developments in Psychopharmacology

Since the 1970s, developments in psychopharmacology, including interventions for children and adolescents, have been occurring at an accelerating pace. For example, in the treatment of ADHD, a variety of stimulants with differing durations of effect are now available. Similarly, for
the treatment of anxiety, depression, and obsessive–compulsive behaviors, a wide range of medications that act as selective serotonin reuptake
inhibitors (SSRIs) have been produced (Brown & Sawyer, 1998).

The assessment of a child's psychological and educational functioning generally is critical in making a determination about whether to use
psychotropic medications (Phelps, Brown, & Power, 2002). The effectiveness of pharmacological interventions has been shown to vary as a
function of specific child characteristics and whether medication is used
separately or in combination with psychosocial interventions (MTA Cooperative Group, 1999; Pelham et al., 1993). For these reasons, collaboration between prescribing physicians, mental healthcare specialists, and
educators is recommended to determine whether medication is indicated, and whether it should be used separately or in combination with a
psychosocial intervention (Phelps et al., 2002).

Pharmacological treatments typically are used to address children's
problems in multiple settings, including home and school. Because it is
not possible to know a priori whether and how a child will respond to
medication, it is important that potentially beneficial and adverse effects
be monitored carefully (Brown & Sawyer, 1998). In response to this

need, multimethod assessment protocols involving informant reports from parents, teachers, and children, as well as direct observations of behavior, have been developed (e.g., DuPaul & Barkley, 1993; Gadow, 1993). The effective management of children using medication typically requires close collaboration among healthcare professionals, families, and school professionals to determine beneficial and adverse effects across multiple systems and domains of functioning (DuPaul & Stoner, 1994; Power, Atkins, Osborne, & Blum, 1994).

Research Documenting the School Problems of Children with Chronic Illnesses

Research conducted on children with chronic illnesses has documented that these individuals often experience impairments in multiple settings, including the school. For instance, children with symptomatic HIV infection commonly manifest neuropsychological impairments that can be progressive or static in nature. These deficits, in turn, may be associated with significant developmental delays and/or learning disorders. In addition, children with symptomatic HIV frequently manifest behavioral and social problems in response to their neurological impairments and/or the psychological problems that may arise in coping with this condition (Wolters, Brouwers, & Moss, 1995). The neurological deficits and psychosocial problems encountered by children with HIV place them at risk for significant impairments in school, community, and family settings. Research with this population has highlighted the need for a comprehensive approach to intervention that addresses their needs in each setting (Landau, Pryor, & Haefli, 1995).

Advancements in research related to children with cancer also has highlighted the need for a multisystemic approach to care. Although the presence of childhood cancer in itself does not increase the risk for psychopathology, it is clear that this illness has a significant emotional and social impact on the child and family, and that the disease can influence functioning in peer groups and in school (Kazak, 2001). In addition, those forms of cancer involving the central nervous system, either because of the illness itself or through its treatment, can have a significant effect on cognitive functioning and academic performance (Armstrong, Blumberg, & Toledano, 1999; Mulhern, 1994).

Emergence of Ecological/Systems Psychology

According to ecological/systems psychology, the behavior of an individual profoundly influences and is influenced by the behavior of every other person in the system (Hobbs, 1966). The behavior of each member of a system is designed to promote the survival and to support the operation of the entire system (Bateson, 1972). Ecological/systems psychology most often has been applied to understand the functioning of children in the family system. The functioning of a child in a family determines and is determined by multiple factors, including the parents' marital relationship, the quality of the parent–child relationships, and the quality of the sibling relationships (Minuchin, Rosman, & Baker, 1978).

Ecological/systems psychology also has been applied to other systems, including the school and healthcare network, and this approach has been used to analyze relationship patterns among systems (Power & Bartholomew, 1987). Bronfenbrenner's (1979) social-ecological model of development, in particular, has provided a broad conceptualization of ecological/systems theory that accounts for the multiple contexts in which children develop. According to this model, each system in a child's life (e.g., family, peer group, school, and healthcare services) is linked with one or more other systems to form a network of interconnected systems or mesosystems. Figure 1.1 illustrates interconnections among the family, school, healthcare, and mental healthcare systems that can have a significant impact on the developing child. The child's functioning in each context influences and is influenced by his or her functioning in the other contexts. Moreover, functioning in each system is highly responsive to the quality of the mesosystemic relationship. For example, research has shown that academic and social performance in school is strongly affected by family involvement in education and a collaborative family–school relationship (Christenson & Sheridan, 2001; Comer, Hayes, Joyner, & Ben-Avie, 1996; Pianta & Walsh, 1996). Similarly, coping with chronic illnesses and mental health disorders can be improved by building collaborative linkages among the family, school, healthcare system, and mental healthcare system (Kazak & Simms, 1996; Logan & King, 2001; Power et al., 1994). The emergence of ecological/systems psychology since the 1960s has further affirmed the critical importance of understanding how children develop within multiple contexts and creating effective connections among the major systems in which children function.

Emphasis on a Positive Approach to Psychology

In psychology, there has been increasing concern about the field's reliance on a deficit-oriented, problem reduction model as a foundation for practice and research (Fantuzzo, Coolahan, & Weiss, 1997). A deficit-oriented model, at best, can provide only a science related to intervention, because there is an implicit assumption that a person must have a problem for the model to be applicable. Although the medical model purports to promote

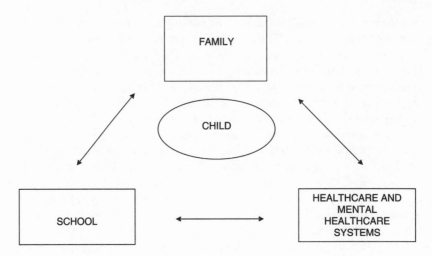

FIGURE 1.1. The development of the child is strongly influenced by interactions among the family, school, healthcare, and mental healthcare systems.

prevention efforts, the focus is on identifying warning signs of pathology and reducing risk with early intervention. With the medical model, the goal is to treat disorder or risk of disorder, which is an approach that may fail to produce outcomes that are truly desirable for people. Furthermore, a deficit orientation does not address the needs of a large segment of society that generally leads happy, productive lives and would like even more fulfillment (Seligman & Csikszentmihalyi, 2000).

In response to concerns about the medical model, an alternative model has been evolving that focuses on the assets of individuals and the systems in which they operate, and that builds the capacity of systems to promote healthy development (Cicchetti, Rappaport, Sandler, & Weissberg, 2000; Cowen, 2000; Frederickson, 2001). In addressing the needs of individuals with coping problems, this positive approach to psychology asserts the importance of identifying protective factors that promote resilient behavior and healthy development in addition to risk factors that are predictive of pathology (Masten, 2001). Furthermore, this approach addresses the needs of the healthy individual who seeks a more fulfilling and productive life. This asset-focused, resource-building approach provides a useful framework for a science of prevention designed to promote human development and healthy lifestyles, in addition to addressing the needs of individuals with emerging evidence of pathology (Seligman & Csikszentmihalyi, 2000).

RESPONDING CREATIVELY TO REFORMS

Social and political reforms, as well as advancements in pediatrics, psychology, and education, have created the need for professionals to serve as leaders in linking systems of care to develop intervention and prevention programs for children and their families (Power, Heathfield, McGoey, & Blum, 1999). Within the field of psychology, several specialties have emerged to address the needs of children and adolescents, including pediatric psychology, school psychology, clinical child psychology, community psychology, and family psychology. Each of these specialties has numerous assets to integrate systems of care in addressing the health needs of children. However, each specialty encounters several limitations in responding to the challenges of reform. The following is a description of the strengths and limitations of two specialties in psychology committed to the provision of healthcare services across systems of care, school psychology and pediatric psychology (see Table 1.2 for an outline of strengths and limitations of each of these subgroups of psychology). Although other child-oriented specialties are also strongly committed to the promotion of children's health, the areas of pediatric and school psychology are highlighted to illustrate how subgroups within child-oriented psychology complement each other and can benefit from engaging in a partnership. It should be noted that school psychology, as it is now being conceptualized by its leaders, is focused on promoting the cognitive, social, emotional, and physical development of children by building the capacity of the school to educate children and by promoting collaborations among the school, family, and community (Ysseldyke et al., 1997). Likewise, pediatric psychology, with its strong roots in clinical child, developmental, and health psychology, is focused on addressing the physical, cognitive, social, and emotional development of children in families and other systems as they relate to issues of health and illness (La Greca & Hughes, 1999; Roberts & McNeal, 1995; Spirito et al., in press).

Contributions from School Psychology

School psychologists are uniquely positioned to respond to reforms related to healthcare because of the emphasis placed on providing intervention and prevention services for children with or at risk for health problems in schools (Dryfoos, 1994). By virtue of their positions in school settings, school psychologists are in an optimal situation to collaborate with school professionals, such as guidance counselors, school nurses, and special education and general education teachers, in developing programs to address the health needs of students.

TABLE 1.2. Strengths and Limitations of School Psychology and Pediatric Psychology in Linking Systems of Care to Address Children's Health Issues

Strengths	Limitations
School psychology	
Situated in schools	Lack of training about illness
Emphasis on data-based decision making	Lack of training related to health systems
Training in functional behavioral assessment	Limited expertise in collaborating with physicians
Expertise promoting family–school collaboration	Primary focus on schools, not community
Expertise working in interdisciplinary teams	Lack of training related to prevention
Pediatric psychology	
Advanced training related to illness	Limited understanding of schools
Expertise regarding medical and psychosocial interventions for illness	Limited understanding of children's functioning in community settings
Understanding of health systems	Lack of focus on prevention
Expertise collaborating with physicians and allied health providers	Lack of training in school consultation
Expertise promoting collaboration between health and family systems	Lack of expertise coordinating school, family, and healthcare systems

The training of school psychologists has prepared them, at least partially, to address the needs of children with health difficulties. The field of school psychology underwent a process of internal reform in the 1980s that shifted the emphasis of the field from assessment for special education disability to intervention for children with or at risk for academic and social problems (Reschly & Ysseldyke, 1995). Although testing activities still consume a high proportion of their time (Reschly & Wilson, 1995), school psychologists are being prepared for roles related to intervention and outcome evaluation and are working to expand their roles in schools to include these activities (Ysseldyke et al., 1997). Relatedly, school psychology has increasingly emphasized the importance of functional behavioral assessment in developing educational and behavioral programs for children, including those with chronic illnesses and mental health disorders (DuPaul & Ervin, 1996; McComas & Mace, 2000). In addition, many school psychologists have been trained to conduct ecological assessments of systems and to promote collaboration between systems, particularly the family and school (Power & Bartholomew, 1987; Sheridan, Kratochwill, & Bergan, 1996), as well as the school and the mental healthcare systems (Reeder et al., 1997). Furthermore, school psychologists have considerable training and expertise in working with interdisciplinary teams to conduct diagnostic assessments and design intervention strategies.

Despite these assets, school psychology as a profession has been limited with regard to the contributions it has been able to make in the management and prevention of health problems. Although school psychologists typically receive training in child psychopathology, they lack training in the areas of acute and chronic illness. School psychology training emphasizes the importance of linking systems of care, but school psychologists have limited training in working with the healthcare system and collaborating with pediatric care providers (HaileMariam, Bradley-Johnson, & Johnson, 2002; Power et al., 1994). Even though school psychologists have important positions in community-based settings, they tend to focus exclusively on school issues. Their work generally does not extend into the community and often fails to link systems of care for children in the neighborhoods served by their schools (Nastasi, 2000; Power, 2000). Furthermore, despite the fact that the school has many resources for supporting prevention and health promotion activities, school psychologists have limited expertise in these areas and often do not have the opportunity to capitalize on the school's assets related to prevention because of systemic demands for the completion of service-related activities (Power, 2000; Short & Talley, 1997).

Contributions from Pediatric Psychology

Pediatric psychologists are uniquely trained to address the health needs of children. These psychologists have advanced training that pertains to medical conditions and the challenges children and their families experience in coping with acute and chronic illnesses. Pediatric psychologists generally base their research and practice on a biopsychosocial model, which recognizes that behavior is determined by a complex transaction of biological, psychological, and social factors, and that a multimodal intervention program, including medical and psychosocial treatments, is often needed to achieve successful outcomes (Roberts & McNeal, 1995).

Pediatric psychologists have expertise regarding a wide range of medical interventions for chronic illnesses and mental health disorders, including surgery, radiation, and chemotherapy for brain tumors (Armstrong & Horn, 1995); insulin and diet management for insulin-dependent diabetes mellitus (Johnson, 1995); medications for the treatment of allergies and asthma (Meyer & Blum, 1997); and psychopharmacological treatments for mental health disorders such as ADHD, tic disorders, anxiety, and depression (Phelps et al., 2002). In addition, pediatric psychologists typically have been trained in the use of psychosocial interventions for the treatment of chronic illnesses and mental health disorders, such as relaxation training for the treatment of abdominal pain (Bursch, Walco, & Zeltzer, 1998), biofeedback for headaches (Allen & Shriver, 1998), urine alarm treatment for nocturnal enuresis (Mellon & Houts, 1995), and cognitive-behavioral interventions for anxiety (Kendall, Krain, & Treadwell, 1999).

Pediatric psychologists generally understand healthcare systems and how to collaborate effectively with physicians and allied health professionals in interdisciplinary teams to address the health needs of children (Drotar, 1995). Furthermore, many pediatric psychologists have been trained to conduct ecological assessments of families and to promote collaborative relationships between healthcare and family systems (Kazak & Simms, 1996).

Despite their vast expertise in addressing the health issues of children and their families, pediatric psychologists are limited in the extent to which they can promote intersystem collaboration and develop a broad continuum of healthcare services, including intervention and prevention programs. Pediatric psychologists generally are limited in their understanding of the school system and methods of consulting with educational professionals. Relatedly, their expertise in promoting collaboration among the health, school, and family systems may be lacking. Although there is increasing emphasis on expanding practice into primary care settings (Strosahl, 1998), pediatric psychologists typically are employed in hospital settings, which places limits on their ability to understand how children function in the community and to promote coordination among community-based systems of care. Furthermore, training pediatric psychologists in methods of prevention has been emphasized by leaders in the field (La Greca & Hughes, 1999; Roberts et al., 1998; Spirito et al., in press), but pediatric psychologists generally focus their practice on intervention and consultation, and engage in a limited amount of prevention activity (Roberts, 1992).

Creating Professional Partnerships: Integrating Pediatric and School Psychology

To respond adaptively to reforms, school and pediatric psychologists must expand their roles and develop new areas of expertise (Power, DuPaul, Shapiro, & Parrish, 1995). School psychologists need to learn more about the management and prevention of health problems and the linking of the healthcare system with the school and family systems (Power, 2002). Similarly, pediatric psychologists must expand their expertise to learn about the school system and methods of integrating the school with the healthcare and family systems to develop intervention and prevention programs.

Responding to the challenges of reform requires a blurring of the traditional distinctions between specialties of child psychology (La Greca & Hughes, 1999). School psychologists increasingly need to learn about pediatric (and clinical child) psychology, and pediatric psychologists need to learn more about school psychology (Power, Shapiro, & DuPaul, in press). In addition, both groups need to expand their learning to include family and community psychology.

Although cross-fertilization among child psychology specialties is needed, the identities of each subgroup can be, and perhaps should be, preserved. School psychologists can expand their roles but continue to focus primarily on improving instructional outcomes by working in educational settings. For school psychologists, the primary purpose of focusing on the healthcare system is to promote the cognitive and social development of each child. Pediatric psychologists can expand the scope of their activities but continue to focus on improving healthcare outcomes through their work in medical settings. For pediatric psychologists, the primary purpose of focusing on the school system is to promote the healthy functioning of children throughout the day and across settings.

Although the roles of school and pediatric psychologists may continue to differ in important ways, there will in all likelihood be considerable overlap. Pediatric psychologists have much to offer in the development and evaluation of school-based health promotion projects, and school psychologists can contribute significantly to the creation of school integration and reintegration initiatives based in healthcare settings. Ongoing collaboration between specialties is essential to avoid counterproductive competition. Maintaining a focus on the common goal of meeting the needs of children and families by responding creatively to national reforms will help to avoid pointless competition and foster productive new partnerships.

As indicated earlier, pediatric and school psychology are not the only child-oriented specialties dedicated to the healthy development of children in multiple contexts. Clinical child, community, and family psychology, among other child-oriented specialties in psychology, clearly are invested in the promotion of children's health in families, schools, and community settings. Likewise, psychology is certainly not the only discipline focused on promoting the integration of community-based systems of care. Primary care health providers, psychiatrists, nurses, and social workers, among others, are committed to very similar goals. Establishing partnerships with professionals from these disciplines is critical for child-oriented psychologists to be effective in linking systems to manage health problems and to promote healthy behaviors for all children and their families.

Through the development of partnerships across disciplines and systems, psychologists and other healthcare providers are able to respond to the challenges presented by children like Sherri, the child described at the beginning of this chapter. In collaboration with the family, school team, and neighborhood leaders, these professionals are in a position to facilitate the comprehensive integration of these children into the school and community.

REFERENCES

Adelman, H. S. (1996). Restructuring educational support services and integrating community resources: Beyond the full service school model. *School Psychology Review, 25*, 431–445.

Adelman, H. S., & Taylor, L. (1998). Mental health in schools: Moving forward. *School Psychology Review, 27*, 175–190.

Allen, K. D., & Shriver, M. (1998). Role of parent mediated pain behavior management strategies in biofeedback treatment of childhood migraine. *Behavior Therapy, 29*, 477–490.

Armstrong, F. D., Blumberg, M. J., & Toledano, S. R. (1999). Neurobehavioral issues in childhood cancer. *School Psychology Review, 28*, 194–203.

Armstrong, F. D., & Horn, M. (1995). Educational issues in childhood cancer. *School Psychology Quarterly, 10*, 292–304.

Bateson, G. (1972). *Steps to an ecology of mind*. New York: Ballantine.

Bickman, L., & Rog, D. J. (Eds.). (1995). *Children's mental health services: Research, policy, and evaluation* (Vol. 1). Thousand Oaks, CA: Sage.

Bronfenbrenner, U. (1979). *The ecology of human development*. Cambridge, MA: Harvard University Press.

Brown, R. T., & Sawyer, M. G. (1998). *Medications for school-age children: Effects on learning and behavior*. New York: Guilford Press.

Bursch, B., Walco, G. A., & Zeltzer, L. (1998). Clinical assessment and management of chronic pain and pain-associated disability syndrome. *Developmental and Behavioral Pediatrics, 19*, 45–53.

Christenson, S. L., & Sheridan, S. M. (2001). *Schools and families: Creating essential connections for learning*. New York: Guilford Press.

Cicchetti, D., Rappaport, J., Sandler, I., & Weissberg, R. P. (Eds.). (2000). *The promotion of wellness in children and adolescents*. Washington, DC: Child Welfare League of America Press.

Comer, J. P., Haynes, N. M., Joyner, E. T., & Ben-Avie, M. (1996). *Rallying the whole village: The Comer process for reforming education*. New York: Teachers College Press.

Cowen, E. L. (2000). Psychological wellness: Some hopes for the future. In D. Cicchetti, J. Rappaport, I. Sandler, & R. P. Weissberg (Eds.), *The promotion of wellness in children and adolescents* (pp. 477–503). Washington, DC: Child Welfare League of America Press.

Creer, T. L., & Bender, B. G. (1995). Pediatric asthma. In M. C. Roberts (Ed.), *Handbook of pediatric psychology* (2nd ed., pp. 219–240). New York: Guilford Press.

Dowrick, P. W., Power, T. J., Manz, P. H., Ginsburg-Block, M., Leff, S. S., & Rupnow, S. K. (2001). Community responsiveness: Examples from under-resourced urban schools. *Journal of Intervention and Prevention in the Community, 21,* 71–90.

Drotar, D. (1995). *Consulting with pediatricians: Psychological perspectives.* New York: Plenum Press.

Dryfoos, J. G. (1994). *Full-service schools: A revolution in health and social services for children, youth, and families.* San Francisco: Jossey-Bass.

DuPaul, G. J., & Barkley, R. A. (1993). The utility of behavioral methodology in medication treatment of children with attention deficit hyperactivity disorder. *Behavior Therapy, 24,* 47–66.

DuPaul, G. J., & Ervin, R. A. (1996). Functional assessment of behaviors related to attention-deficit/hyperactivity disorder. *Behavior Therapy, 27,* 601–622.

DuPaul, G. J., & Stoner, G. (1994). *ADHD in the schools: Assessment and intervention strategies.* New York: Guilford Press.

Fantuzzo, J., Coolahan, K. C., & Weiss, A. D. (1997). Resiliency partnership-directed intervention: Enhancing the social competencies of preschool victims of physical abuse by developing peer resources and community strengths. In D. Cicchetti & S. L. Toth (Eds.), *Rochester Symposium on Developmental Psychopathology: Vol. 8. Developmental perspectives on trauma: Theory, research, and intervention* (pp. 463–489). Rochester, NY: University of Rochester Press.

Fantuzzo, J. W., & Mohr, W. (2000). Pursuit of wellness in Head Start: Making beneficial connections for children and families. In D. Cicchetti, J. Rapapport, I. Sandler, & R. Weissberg (Eds.), *The promotion of wellness in children and adolescents* (pp. 341–369). Thousand Oaks, CA: Sage.

Farmer, J. E., Clippard, D. S., Luehr-Wiemann, Y., Wright, E., & Owings, S. (1997). Assessing children with traumatic brain injury during rehabilitation: Promoting school and community reentry. In E. D. Bigler, E. Clark, & J. E. Farmer (Eds.), *Childhood traumatic brain injury: Diagnosis, assessment, and intervention* (pp. 33–62). Austin, TX: Pro-Ed.

Fredrickson, B. L. (2001). The role of positive emotions in positive psychology: The broaden-and-build theory of positive emotions. *American Psychologist, 56,* 218–226.

Gadow, K. D. (1993). A school-based medication evaluation program. In J. L. Matson (Ed.), *Handbook of hyperactivity in children* (pp. 186–219). Boston: Allyn & Bacon.

Gittelsohn, J., Toporoff, E. G., Story, M., Evans, M., Anliker, J., Davis, S., Sharma, A., & White, J. (1999). Food perceptions and dietary behavior of American-Indian children, their caregivers, and educators: Formative assessment findings from Pathways. *Journal of Nutrition Education, 31,* 2–13.

Goals 2000: Educate America Act. (1994). U.S. Congress, Public Law 103–227.

HaileMariam, A., Bradley-Johnson, S., Johnson, C. M. (2002). Pediatricians' preferences for ADHD information from schools. *School Psychology Review, 31,* 94–105.

Hobbs, N. (1966). Helping disturbed children: Psychological and ecological strategies. *American Psychologist, 21,* 1105–1115.

Individuals with Disabilities Education Act—Amendments of 1997. (1997). U.S. Congress, Public Law 101–476; amended by Public Law 105–17.

Johnson, S. B. (1995). Insulin-dependent diabetes mellitus in childhood. In M. C. Roberts (Ed.), *Handbook of pediatric psychology* (2nd ed., pp. 263–285). New York: Guilford Press.

Kazak, A. E. (2001). Comprehensive care for children with cancer and their families: A social ecological framework guiding research, practice and policy. *Children's Services: Social Policy, Research and Practice, 4,* 217–233.

Kazak, A. E., & Simms, S. (1996). Children with life-threatening illnesses: Psychological difficulties and interpersonal relationships. In F. Kaslow (Ed.), *Handbook of relational diagnosis and dysfunctional family patterns* (pp. 225–238). New York: Wiley.

Kazdin, A. E., Holland, L., & Crowley, M. (1997). Family experience of barriers to treatment and premature termination from child therapy. *Journal of Consulting and Clinical Psychology, 65,* 453–463.

Kendall, P. C., Krain, A., & Treadwell, K. (1999). Generalized anxiety disorders. In R. H. Ammerman, M. Hersen, & C. G. Last (Eds.), *Handbook of prescriptive treatments for children and adolescents* (pp. 155–171). Boston: Allyn & Bacon.

Knoff, H. M. (1996). The interface of school, community, and healthcare reform: Organizational directions toward effective services for children and youth. *School Psychology Review, 25,* 446–464.

Kolbe, L. J., Collins, J., & Cortese, P. (1997). Building the capacity of schools to improve the health of the nation: A call for assistance from psychologists. *American Psychologist, 52,* 256–265.

La Greca, A. M., & Hughes, J. N. (1999). United we stand, divided we fall: The education and training of clinical child psychologists. *Journal of Clinical Child Psychology, 28,* 435–447.

Landau, S., Pryor, J. B., & Haefli, K. (1995). Pediatric HIV: School-based sequelae and curricular interventions for infection prevention and social acceptance. *School Psychology Review, 24,* 213–229.

Leff, S. S., Power, T. J., Manz, P. H., Costigan, T. E., & Nabors, L. A. (2001). School-based aggression prevention programs for young children: Current status and implications for violence prevention. *School Psychology Review, 30,* 344–362.

Logan, D. E., & King, C. A. (2001). Parental facilitation of adolescent mental health service utilization: A conceptual and empirical review. *Clinical Psychology Science and Practice, 8,* 319–333.

Masten, A. S. (2001). Ordinary magic: Resilience processes in development. *American Psychologist, 56,* 227–238.

McComas, J. J., & Mace, F. C. (2000). Theory and practice in conducting functional analysis. In E. S. Shapiro & T. R. Kratochwill (Eds.), *Behavioral assess-*

ment in schools: Theory, research, and clinical foundations (2nd ed., pp. 78–103). New York: Guilford Press.

McMiller, W. P., & Weisz, J. R. (1996). Help-seeking preceding mental health clinic intake among African-American, Latino, and Caucasian youths. *Journal of the American Academy of Child and Adolescent Psychiatry, 35,* 1086–1094.

Mellon, M., & Houts, A. (1995). Elimination disorders. In R. Ammerman & M. Hersen (Eds.), *Handbook of child behavior therapy in the psychiatric setting* (pp. 341–365). New York: Wiley.

Meyer, G. A., & Blum, N. J. (1997). Allergies and asthma. In G. G. Bear, K. M. Minke, & A. Thomas (Eds.), *Children's needs: II. Development, problems, and alternatives.* Washington, DC: National Association of School Psychologists.

Minuchin, S., Rosman, B. L., & Baker, L. (1978). *Psychosomatic families.* Cambridge, MA: Harvard University Press.

MTA Cooperative Group. (1999). Mediators and moderators of treatment response for children with attention-deficit/hyperactivity disorder: The Multimodal Treatment Study of Children with Attention Deficit Hyperactivity Disorder Study. *Archives of General Psychiatry, 56,* 1088–1096.

Mulhern, P. K. (1994). Neuropsychological late effects. In D. J. Bearison & R. K. Mulhern (Eds.), *Pediatric psychooncology: Psychological perspectives on children with cancer* (pp. 99–121). New York: Oxford University Press.

Nastasi, B. K. (2000). School psychologists as health-care providers in the 21st century: Conceptual framework, professional identity, and professional practice. *School Psychology Review, 29,* 540–554.

Nastasi, B. K., Varjas, K., Schensul, S. L., Silva, K. T., Schensul, J. J., & Ratnayake, P. (2000). The participatory intervention model: A framework for conceptualizing and promoting intervention acceptability. *School Psychology Quarterly, 15,* 207–232.

Pavuluri, M. N., Luk, S. L., & Mcgee, R. (1996). Help-seeking for behavior problems by parents of preschool children: A community study. *Journal of the American Academy of Child and Adolescent Psychiatry, 35,* 215–222.

Pelham, W. E., Carlson, C., Sams, S. E., Vallano, G., Dixon, J., & Hoza, B. (1993). Separate and combined effects of methylphenidate and behavior modification on boys with attention deficit-hyperactivity disorder in the classroom. *Journal of Consulting and Clinical Psychology, 61,* 506–515.

Phelps, L., Brown, R. T., & Power, T. J. (2002). *Pediatric psychopharmacology: Combining medical and psychosocial interventions.* Washington, DC: American Psychological Association.

Pianta, R. C., & Walsh, D. (1996). *High risk children in the schools: Creating sustaining relationships.* New York: Routledge.

Power, T. J. (2000). Commentary: The school psychologist as community-focused, public health professional: Emerging challenges and implications for training. *School Psychology Review, 29,* 557–559.

Power, T. J. (2002). Preparing school psychologists as interventionists and preventionists. In M. R. Shinn, H. M. Walker, & G. Stoner (Eds.), *Interventions for academic and behavior problems: II. Preventive and remedial approaches* (pp. 1047–1065). Bethesda, MD: National Association of School Psychologists.

Power, T. J., Atkins, M. S., Osborne, M. L., & Blum, N. J. (1994). The school psychologist as manager of programming for ADHD. *School Psychology Review, 23*, 279–291.

Power, T. J., & Bartholomew, K. L. (1987). Family–school relationship patterns: An ecological assessment. *School Psychology Review, 14*, 222–229.

Power, T. J., DuPaul, G. J., Shapiro, E. S., & Parrish, J. M. (1995). Pediatric school psychology: The emergence of a subspecialty. *School Psychology Review, 24*, 244–257.

Power, T. J., Heathfield, L., McGoey, K., & Blum, N. J. (1999). Managing and preventing chronic health problems: School psychology's role. *School Psychology Review, 28*, 251–263.

Power, T. J., Manz, P. H., & Leff, S. S. (in press). Training for effective practice in the schools. In M. Weist, S. Evans, & N. Tashman (Eds.), *School mental health handbook*. Norwell, MA: Kluwer Academic/Plenum Publishers.

Power, T. J., Shapiro, E. S., & DuPaul, G. J. (2001). *Preparing leaders in child psychology for the 21st century: Linking systems of care to manage and prevent health problems*. Manuscript submitted for publication.

Reeder, G. D., Maccow, G. C., Shaw, S. R., Swerdlik, M. E., Horton, C. B., & Foster, P. (1997). School psychologists and full service schools: Partnerships with medical, mental health, and social services. *School Psychology Review, 26*, 603–621.

Reschly, D. J., & Wilson, M. S. (1995). School psychology practitioners and faculty: 1986 to 1991–92—Trends in demographics, roles, satisfaction, and system reform. *School Psychology Review, 24*, 62–80.

Reschly, D. J., & Ysseldyke, J. E. (1995). School psychology paradigm shift. In A. Thomas & J. Grimes (Eds.), *Best practices in school psychology—III* (pp. 17–31). Washington, DC: National Association of School Psychologists.

Roberts, M. C. (1992). *Vale dictum*: An editor's view of the field of pediatric psychology and its journal. *Journal of Pediatric Psychology, 17*, 785–805.

Roberts, M. C., Carlson, C., Erickson, M., Friedman, R., La Greca, A., Lemanek, K., Russ, S., Schroeder, C., Vargas, L., & Wohlford, P. (1998). A model for training psychologists to provide services for children and adolescents. *Professional Psychology: Research and Practice, 29*, 293–299.

Roberts, M. C., & Hurley, L. K. (1997). *Managing managed care*. New York: Plenum Press.

Roberts, M. C., & McNeal, R. E. (1995). Historical and conceptual foundations of pediatric psychology. In M. C. Roberts (Ed.), *Handbook of pediatric psychology* (2nd ed., pp. 3–18). New York: Guilford Press.

Seligman, M. E. P., & Csikszentmihalyi, M. (2000). Positive psychology. *American Psychologist, 55*, 5–14.

Shaffer, D., Fisher, P., Dulcan, M. K., Davies, M., Piacentini, J., Schwab-Stone, M. E., Lahey, B., Bourdon, K., Jensen, P., Bird, H., Canino, G., & Regier, D. (1996). The NIMHD Diagnostic Interview Schedule for Children Version 2.3 (DISC-2.3): Description, acceptability, prevalence rates, and performance in the MECA Study (Methods for the Epidemiology of Child and Adolescent

Mental Disorders Study). *Journal of the American Academy of Child and Adolescent Psychiatry, 35*, 865–877.

Sheridan, S. M., Kratochwill, T. R., & Bergan, J. R. (1996). *Conjoint behavioral consultation: A procedural manual.* New York: Plenum Press.

Short, R. J., & Talley, R. C. (1997). Rethinking psychology in the schools: Implications of recent national policy. *American Psychologist, 52*, 234–240.

Spirito, A., Brown, R. T., D'Angelo, E., Delameter, A., Rodrique, J., & Siegel, L. (in press). Recommendations for the training of pediatric psychologists. *Journal of Pediatric Psychology.*

Strosahl, K. (1998). Integrating behavioral health and primary care services: The primary mental healthcare model. In A. Blount (Ed.), *Integrated primary care* (pp. 139–166). New York: Norton.

Talley, R. C., & Short, R. J. (1995). *School health: Psychology's role: A report to the nation.* Washington, DC: American Psychological Association.

Tharinger, D. J., Bricklin, P., Johnson, N. F., Paster, V., Lambert, N. M., Feshbach, N., Oakland, T. D., & Sanchez, W. (1996). Education reform: Challenges for psychology and psychologists. *Professional Psychology: Research and Practice, 27*, 24–33.

Troiano, R. P., Flegal, K. M., Kuczmarski, R. J., Campbell, S. M., & Johnson, C. L. (1995). Overweight and obesity prevalence trends for children and adolescents. *Archives of Pediatric and Adolescent Medicine, 149*, 1085–1091.

U.S. Department of Health and Human Services. (1999). *Mental health: A report of the Surgeon General.* Rockville, MD: U.S. Department of Health and Human Services, Substance Abuse and Mental Health Administration, Center for Mental healthcare services, National Institutes of Health, National Institute of Mental Health.

U.S. Department of Health and Human Services. (2001). *Mental health: Culture, race, and ethnicity: A supplement to mental health: A report of the Surgeon General.* Rockville, MD: U.S. Department of Health and Human Services, Substance Abuse and Mental Health Administration, Center for Mental healthcare services, National Institutes of Health, National Institute of Mental Health.

Wolters, P. L., Brouwers, P., & Moss, H. A. (1995). Pediatric HIV disease: Effect on cognition, learning, and behavior. *School Psychology Quarterly, 10*, 305–328.

Ysseldyke, J., Dawson, P., Lehr, C., Reschly, D., Reynolds, M., & Telzrow, C. (1997). *School psychology: A blueprint for training and practice II.* Bethesda, MD: National Association of School Psychologists.

CHAPTER 2

Addressing Healthcare Issues across Settings

Children's healthcare issues encompass the broad range of contexts in which children function, including families, schools, healthcare settings, and formal and informal neighborhood agencies. The healthcare reform movement has focused attention on the need to create a service delivery system that includes all of these contexts. In general, there have been few attempts to provide an integrative perspective on the capacities of these different settings to provide care for children with a wide variety of health conditions. In this chapter, we examine factors that have an impact on service delivery, and the assets and limitations of providing healthcare in diverse settings.

Reforms in healthcare, largely driven by economic factors, and including the managed care movement, have had dramatic effects on the provision of healthcare services for children and their families (Roberts & Hurley, 1997). In comparing families today with those of the previous generation, healthcare for many may be more expensive, less available, and more uncertain. Of course, in some cases, managed care has facilitated the delivery of preventive and routine healthcare, often at a lower cost to families. However, in the case of children with complex pediatric healthcare needs, the managed care system often is viewed skeptically in its delivery of care; that is, providing care optimally matched to the needs of the child and family during periods of acute and chronic healthcare needs, and doing so in a manner that is cost-effective while also achieving patient and family satisfaction, has been challenging (Drotar & Zagorski, 2001).

It is unfortunate and ironic that access to care is restricted at a time when achievements in medicine have provided new, life-saving, and life-enhancing treatments. There are many examples of these accomplishments in pediatrics. A few of the more evident achievements include the improved survival of premature very low birth-weight infants; more aggressive and successful treatments that have improved survival for children with cancer; increased development of organ transplantation protocols for children with severe heart, lung, liver and kidney disease; and medication regimens that sustain life for children with HIV/AIDS. Although these treatments save lives, each has significant psychosocial morbidity attached to it. The long-term physical and mental disabilities associated with low birth weight, for example, can impact the child's life and that of the family in dramatic fashion. As another example, the long-term healthcare needs of a child with an organ transplant are difficult to meet when transplantation sequelae may include medications with unpleasant side effects, repeated surgeries, and/or adaptations in physical activity and lifestyle. Models of service delivery to address the biopsychosocial needs of children with complex health conditions clearly have not kept pace with the enormous advancements in medicine.

One very clear change that has occurred in response to healthcare reform is the amount and nature of care provided in hospitals. The current healthcare delivery system restricts access to expensive, intensive, hospital-based care. Even when hospital-based services are required and approved, the managed care system restricts the amount of care provided by minimizing the length of inpatient hospital stays, and limiting the type and amount of specialized service rendered (Roberts & Hurley, 1997). A major impact of this movement has been to increase the responsibility of families and community-based providers, including primary pediatric care practitioners and school professionals, for the delivery of health services (Brown & Freeman, 2002). At the same time, community providers struggle with ways of responding to increased demands for services.

Reforms in healthcare also have been spawned by concerns about variable access to services. Families of low-income status from urban as well as rural settings, and particularly those of minority backgrounds, are much more likely to have problems accessing services than families in more advantaged circumstances (U.S. Department of Health and Human Services, 2001). Even when services are available, they may not be rendered in a culturally sensitive manner by providers who are well-trained, experienced, and committed to working with children and families.

This chapter considers the strengths and limitations of a range of settings in which healthcare is currently provided, highlighting the need for coordination of health services among systems to address the complex health needs of children and families. In addition, this chapter discusses factors that have an impact on service provision in a variety of settings, including regional and community hospitals, community-based primary care practices, schools, neighborhood agencies and organizations, and the home.

DIVERSE SETTINGS FOR HEALTHCARE

Healthcare services are being delivered in multiple settings. Each venue is associated with a number of strengths and limitations. The following is a description of the assets and disadvantages associated with the provision of healthcare in alternative settings. Table 2.1 provides a comparison of three of these settings (i.e., hospital, primary care, and school) with regard to the following dimensions of healthcare: (1) expertise of providers, (2) sophistication of medical technology, (3) capacity to address severe health conditions, (4) availability of interdisciplinary collaboration, (5) opportunities for family involvement and collaboration, (6) potential for preventive care, (7) opportunities for providing assessment and intervention in naturalistic settings, (8) potential for culturally sensitive care, (9) financial costs, and (10) accessibility of intervention.

TABLE 2.1. Benefits and Limitations of Hospital Care, Primary Care, and School-Based Healthcare

Variables	Hospital care	Primary care	School-based services
Level of medical expertise	High	Moderate	Generally low and variable
Sophistication of technology	High	Moderate	Generally low
Capacity to address severe conditions	High	Low to moderate	Low
Opportunities for interdisciplinary care	High among health staff	Generally low	High among educational staff
Opportunities for family involvement	Low to moderate	High	High
Accessibility of services	Generally low	High	High
Opportunities for prevention work	Low	High	High
Potential for naturalistic intervention	Low	Low to moderate	High
Potential for culturally responsive care	Low to moderate	High	High
Financial costs for services	Generally high	Low to moderate	Low to moderate

Hospital-Based Care

Hospitals employ healthcare professionals with a high level of expertise and have sophisticated medical technology available to diagnose and treat medical disorders. These settings generally have the capacity to address medical conditions with a moderate to high level of severity (e.g., cancer, heart disease). Hospitals can differ markedly in the degree of specialization and technology provided. Community hospitals tend to have a somewhat limited range or number of specialists available and a moderate level of technology, whereas tertiary care centers typically have a broad range of specialists and highly sophisticated technology. Hospitals with academic affiliations have as a primary mission basic and applied research to reduce disease and improve health. Academic medical centers are also committed to training, with trainees (e.g., medical residents and fellows) providing care under supervision.

Hospitals typically employ professionals from a variety of allied health professions, including nursing, physical therapy, occupational therapy, respiratory therapy, speech and language pathology, social work, child life, and psychology, providing abundant opportunities for interdisciplinary collaboration (see Drotar, 1995). However, hospitals are limited with regard to educational services and linkages with schools and community-based providers (Drotar & Zagorski, 2001).

Increasingly, hospitals are emphasizing the importance of family-centered care in pediatrics, although access to services for families may be limited, particularly in tertiary care sites. Hospitals focus on addressing the needs of individuals who are ill, and preventive care may be less central to their mission. Because hospitals often are removed from the community, health professionals may be limited with regard to understanding children's functioning in naturalistic contexts and planning interventions that are generalizable to real-life settings. Hospital-based services are relatively expensive, which is necessary to support a large administrative infrastructure, a wide range of medical specialties and allied health professions, malpractice insurance costs, and sophisticated technology.

Primary Care

Primary care providers typically are generalists working in community-based healthcare settings who are knowledgeable about a wide range of health conditions but may lack expertise related to specific illnesses. Primary care practices are equipped with some sophisticated technologies but to a much lesser degree than hospital-based sites. Their capacity to address medical conditions that require a complex treatment regimen is limited. Opportunities for interdisciplinary collaboration generally are lacking, because physicians and nursing staff at several levels (e.g., nurses aides, nurses, nurse practitioners) may be the only professional groups represented. Psychologists have the potential to serve important roles in primary care settings, and pediatric psychologists have identified the integration of psychology into primary care as a priority for the future (Brown & Roberts, 2000). Recently, an increasing number of psychologists have been initiating programs of clinical practice and research in primary care settings to address this need for collaborative care (see the special issue on Pediatric Mental Health Services in Primary Care Settings in *Journal of Pediatric Psychology*, 1999, Vol. 24, No. 5).

The mission of primary care in pediatrics is to address the needs of the developing child, with an appreciation for the family context in which the child functions. Because primary care practices typically are based in the community, access for families generally is quite good. An exception may occur in certain urban and rural communities in which primary care is less available. Primary care practitioners provide services for healthy children, so there is great potential for preventive care. Although primary care sites typically are embedded in the community, they operate to some extent in isolation from the natural settings in which children function (i.e., schools, families, neighborhood organizations). For this reason, opportunities to understand and modify children's behavior in naturalistic contexts may be quite limited. The potential for collaboration with the schools is high, but logistical barriers (e.g., limited time and differences in nomenclature) typically preclude communication between the primary care and educational systems. Similarly, the potential for providing care in a community-responsive, culturally sensitive manner is strong, particularly when they are situated in the neighborhoods in which children reside. However, pediatric care practices may confront the same challenges that schools face when trying to respond to children and families from diverse cultures and socioeconomic groups (see Comer, Haynes, Joyner, & Ben-Avie, 1996).

The managed care movement and other health reforms have ensured that primary care services are affordable for a high percentage of children, although fiscal barriers still preclude adequate care for a sizable minority of children (Roberts & Hurley, 1997). Furthermore, largely because of their accessibility and fiscal affordability, primary care sites have become vital in the screening, assessment, and treatment of a wide range of mental health disorders, including attention-deficit/ hyperactivity disorder (ADHD), anxiety disorders, and mood disorders (Brown & Freeman, 2002; Stancin & Palermo, 1997). The creation and dissemination of the *Diagnostic and Statistical Manual for Primary Care* (DSM-PC) – Child and Adolescent Version (American Academy of Pediatrics, 1996) is a response to the need for mental health screening and diagnostic tools in primary care. In addition, the Bright Futures Program (National Center for Education in Maternal and Child Health, 2000) has been developed in large part to address the need for guidelines in the assessment and treatment of mental health problems in primary care.

School-Based Healthcare

Schools employ professionals with expertise in a wide range of educational and mental healthcare issues, but knowledge about medical issues may be limited. The school nurse is the professional typically designated as the school health expert, although the availability of school nurses can be highly variable. Opportunities for interdisciplinary care are afforded by schools through teams focusing on evaluation and intervention; however, the involvement of external healthcare and mental healthcare professionals on these teams generally is lacking. Schools are embedded in neighborhoods and for that reason can be highly accessible for families and have the potential to provide services in a culturally responsive manner. However, many families feel disconnected from the school and perceive school professionals as unresponsive to family and community needs (Christenson & Sheridan, 2001). Fragmentation between the school and community often is most problematic in low-income neighborhoods in which school staff may not be sufficiently responsive to the needs of families from diverse ethnic and cultural groups (Comer et al., 1996).

Schools provide outstanding opportunities for understanding the functioning of children across multiple domains (academic, adult-oriented social behavior, peer-oriented social behavior) in naturalistic settings (Power & Blom-Hoffman, in press). In addition, schools are a valuable source of normative data for evaluating the functioning of children relative to peers of similar age and gender. Schools are naturally suited to prevention activities, because about 95% of children attend schools, and the mission of the schools is consistent with the promotion of competence and health as opposed to a deficit-focused orientation prevalent in health and mental health clinics (Power & Blom-Hoffman, in press). To the extent that public funds are available through local tax revenues, federal and state educational funding, and Medicaid, the financial cost of health services provided in schools is relatively low.

Healthcare in Other Community-Based Settings

Health and social services may be provided in many other formal and informal settings in the community, including sports and recreational clubs, faith-based organizations, afterschool programs, and welfare-to-work programs (Tucker, 2002). The assets of these settings are their accessibility to families, their responsiveness to the naturalistic patterns of help-seeking behavior represented in the neighborhoods, their potential for understanding and addressing the needs of children and families in real-life contexts, and the extensive opportunities available for health promotion (Benson, 1997). Obvious limitations of these programs include the lack of medical expertise and technology to support health programming, and the lack of resources to track accountability, evaluate outcomes, and ensure high-quality care.

Integrating Systems of Care

Each system of healthcare is associated with numerous assets and limitations for providing health and mental health services for children and their families. Although each system has the potential to be more useful to children, factors intrinsic to each system place severe restrictions on the amount of change that can be expected. For example, hospitals can emphasize the importance of being responsive to families from various cultures, but the need to serve families from many diverse cultures, their distance from the neighborhoods they serve, and the institutionalized environment in which they are based place limits on their ability to be community-responsive. Likewise, schools have the potential to provide helpful services to address the health needs of children and families, but there are substantial limits on the resources that schools can muster to address the complex health needs of children.

For this reason, partnerships across systems are absolutely essential to address the changing health needs of children in a culturally responsive manner. Unfortunately, these systems often work in isolation, and there is limited collaboration among them. Primary care providers and school professionals have limited contact with each other, which deprives each system of the benefits available from collaborating with the other system. Schools often are disconnected from grassroots organizations embedded in the community that have been formed to respond to the help-seeking patterns of residents, resulting in a failure of the schools to be responsive to families, and a failure of the community to benefit from the expertise of the educational staff (Comer et al., 1996).

Creative methods for integrating systems of care need to be developed within each community by those committed to the healthcare of its children. Principal stakeholder groups include hospital- and clinic-based professionals, primary care providers, school personnel, neighborhood-based agency staff, and family members. Psychologists serving the community can be invaluable in facilitating the process of integration and evaluating its progress in a formative manner (Kolbe, Collins, & Cortese, 1997).

FACTORS IMPACTING THE CAPACITY OF COMMUNITY-BASED SYSTEMS

The capacity of the community to address the health needs of children and their families depends on numerous factors, including (1) the medical condition and health needs of the child, (2) the family's psychosocial risk and resilience, (3) collaboration among community-based systems, and (4) help-seeking patterns of the family. The following is a description of each of these factors.

Health Status and Healthcare Needs of the Child

The child's medical condition and the complexity of the intervention regimen to manage the disorder clearly are important in determining the most appropriate healthcare setting. The more complex the condition and its treatments, the more highly specialized the therapeutic environment needs to be. For example, a child with severe heart and lung disease who is preparing for organ transplantation generally is best served in a tertiary-care hospital that has a team of specialists with the expertise to address the complex medical and psychosocial issues faced by the child and family. Alternatively, a child with a disease that typically is less severe, such as asthma, may be treated exclusively in a primary care practice with a focus on the most salient and immediate symptoms of the illness.

Whereas medicine is organized by specific diseases and organ systems, psychological issues tend to be cross-cutting. Thus, in working with children who have pediatric healthcare needs, one must balance disease-specific information with knowledge of how illness and treatment affects children and families in general. In order to do so, a series of general illness/treatment parameters may be identified that can help guide psychosocial care.

One issue is prevalence. From a public health perspective, the more prevalent a disorder, the more important it is to have a broad spectrum of providers available in community settings to address the medical and psychological issues associated with the condition. For example, given the prevalence of asthma, obesity, and diabetes, it is important that professionals knowledgeable about these conditions be available in community settings that are highly accessible to children and families coping with these conditions. Epidemiological data indicate that the prevalence of disorders can change markedly over time. For example, as the prevalence of ADHD and autism increase, the need for community-based systems of care becomes heightened. Furthermore, as more children are cured of cancer, the prevalence of childhood cancer survivors is increasing, which has implications for the care of children in primary care, school, and other community settings. A major challenge faced by the healthcare system is to increase access to services for children and families coping with disorders and illnesses that are relatively prevalent (Brown & Freeman, 2002).

Within most pediatric conditions, there is a spectrum of severity related to the prognosis of the illness and its impact on daily life. It is tempting to think that there is a clear relationship between the severity of the illness, as judged by more objective medical criteria, and psychological adjustment. However, this often is not the case. Indeed, research has shown that subjective appraisal of the impact of a health problem is a more potent predictor of psychological adjustment than medical parameters of severity (Kazak et al., 1998). It also may be the case that there are indirect relationships. In a recent study, sickle-cell disease severity was not related to routine healthcare service utilization but was associated with parental stress (Logan, Radcliffe, & Smith-Whitely, 2002). This highlights an issue that often is misunderstood and can lead to conflict between families and healthcare providers. Specifically, a condition that is prevalent and may not be viewed as severe from a medical perspective may be perceived as serious, disruptive, or threatening to a child and family, possibly resulting in behavior that seems disproportionate to the condition medically.

Two aspects of severity deserve particular attention, that is, the extent to which a condition threatens the child's life, and the neurocognitive impact of the condition. Across a series of studies of different child illnesses, these issues have been shown to be associated with well-being. There is some degree of loss associated with the onset of any serious childhood illness, even if limited to the need to adjust expectations for the child's performance on a short-term basis. However, in the case of life-threatening illness, loss is pervasive and unavoidable. Perhaps for this reason, posttraumatic stress has proven to be a helpful model for understanding the reactions of children and their parents to a life-threatening illness. In studies of children who have survived cancer and organ transplantation, symptoms of posttraumatic stress are reported among children and their parents (e.g., Kazak et al., 1998). Symptoms include primarily intrusive memories about the trauma (e.g., parents recalling when their child was admitted to the intensive care unit; children recalling another child who died), although other symptoms of posttraumatic stress, such as avoidance and physiological arousal, also are common. In addition, illness that impacts neurocognitive functioning generally results in higher levels of child and family distress (Wade et al., 2001; Wade, Taylor, Drotar, Stancin, & Yeates, 1996). These types of illnesses may have salient effects on school functioning, resulting in learning and attention problems, peer relationship difficulties, emotional distress, and poor attendance (see Brown, 1999). Less often appreciated is the extent to which neurocognitive difficulties may affect the child's social and family life, and generate more ongoing distress.

Elevated levels of psychological difficulty frequently are noted in children with pediatric chronic illnesses. However, the literature actually provides little support for elevated levels of psychopathology (Kazak, Rourke, & Crump, in press). There are a couple of complicating factors that have not been well accounted for in the research in this area. One is the process by which social and emotional concerns develop over time. It is possible that factors inherent in the illness generally may be unrelated to psychological disturbance, but the illness serves as a risk factor that can be exacerbated by other problems (e.g., family conflict) and can escalate into more severe difficulties (e.g., increased conflict, family violence, or divorce). Alternatively, a history of behavioral and emotional problems prior to the diagnosis of a pediatric condition can be a risk factor for ongoing concerns. In terms of social relationships, many children with chronic illnesses relate effectively with their peers and show no differences from well-matched controls (e.g., Vannatta, Gertstein, Short, & Noll, 1998). Similarly, the child's maturity and temperament may predict ongoing adjustment or difficulty (Wallander, Hubert, & Varni, 1988). For example, children who have fewer friends, who are more fearful, immature, or hyperactive than others their age, may have difficulty with the challenges faced in treatment.

Risk and Resilience of Families

Families vary tremendously in their capacities and approaches to caring for children with healthcare needs. Some families seem capable of adjusting to serious, chronic illnesses with relatively little overt distress, yet others falter and exhibit symptoms of distress in several family members when confronted with less medically challenging situations. Families also are very complex. How can we tease apart some of the factors that influence family adaptiveness in the face of managing pediatric illness?

Most families of ill children function within normal limits; well-controlled studies repeatedly have shown more similarities than differences between families with and without ill children (Kazak, Rourke, & Crump, in press; Kazak, Segal-Andrews, & Johnson, 1995; Quittner & DiGirolamo, 1998). Most families respond and reorganize competently after the disruptions surrounding, for example, a diagnosis of childhood cancer (Kazak & Simms, 1996; Simms & Kazak, 1998). There is some evidence that those families who may have more difficulty responding to the cancer diagnosis across time can be identified early. In their benchmark longitudinal study of families of children with cancer, Kupst and colleagues (1995) have shown that families with the most difficulty coping at time of diagnosis continue to experience the highest levels of distress, even after treatment ends. The prospective studies of Kazak and colleagues also have shown that parental distress at the time of diagnosis is a significant predictor of ongoing distress (Kazak et al., 1997; Best, Streisand, Catania, & Kazak, 2001). Identifying families at high risk for later disturbances allows for the targeted delivery of preventive interventions aimed at diminishing subsequent distress, as well as reducing existing difficulties.

Our model of risk and resilience among families coping with health problems is guided by our adaptation of the prevention framework outlined by the Institute of Medicine (1994). Because the majority of families are psychologically healthy, albeit distressed, the notion of classifying families by risk is appealing. It provides a model in which services are provided to all families, but with higher levels of care to those families most at risk (see Figure 2.1). In this case, *universal* care is designed to address the reactions of virtually all families of children seeking healthcare. Parents may be anxious, but most are able to cope and adapt with general psychosocial support and attention to anticipated difficulties during treatment. Parents are likely to be able to collaborate with schools in ensuring that their child's healthcare needs are provided for in the school setting.

A smaller set of families requires *selective* care; that is, they present with factors that predispose them to ongoing difficulties. Their coping skills are challenged and may be exceeded. These families are likely to have more difficulty in forming collaborative relationships with schools and in tolerating challenges that are inevitable in coordinating care.

Finally, families falling within the *indicated* realm have several factors suggestive of high risk for ongoing distress, including elevated and persistent anxiety, and other comorbid child and family psychosocial problems. These families generally will benefit from more individualized psychosocial treatment and have already been recognized as needing such care within the educational setting. Consistent with this prevention model, we propose that the largest number of families fall within the universal range, with the smallest number requiring the most intensive psychosocial care (indicated).

Based on a review of the pediatric healthcare literature, several domains of family risk may be identified. For example, single-parent fami-

UNIVERSAL *(largest grp of families)*

Generally well-functioning children and families.
Coping with stressors associated with pediatric illness.
Adequate social support, no evidence of psychopathology or other serious problems.
Likely to be anxious, but parent and child show ability to modulate distress.
Realistic beliefs that are helpful.

Provide general psychosocial assessment and support.
Help families anticipate/prevent further difficulties related to adherence.
Expect course of recovery, coping competently, and improvement in functioning.

SELECTIVE

Some indication of factors that predispose family to risk.
Coping skills may be limited.
Adherence problems possible or likely.
Pile-up of stressors is possible.

More intensive psychosocial support (e.g., groups, programs, assistance
with identified concerns, including adherence) needed.

INDICATED *(smallest #)*

Several high-risk indicators present.
High and persistent anxiety, other psychological difficulties.
Consultation suggested; ongoing escalation is a risk.

FIGURE 2.1. Levels of prevention/intervention for families coping with health conditions. The proportion of families requiring services at each level is progressively smaller across the universal, selected, and indicated levels.

lies have been identified as having higher levels of risk for psychosocial difficulties (Kids Count, 1999). A higher number of siblings also may be associated with greater family stress (Menaghan, 1999; Sameroff, Bartko, Baldwin, Baldwin, & Seifer, 1998).

In general, poverty, particularly in urban settings, is a risk factor for a wide range of psychosocial difficulties (Kids Count, 1999; Black & Krishakumar, 1998). Many families experience changes in their employment and family income at or shortly after diagnosis of a serious pediatric illness. Combined with the sudden increase in healthcare costs and associated expenses (e.g., travel to the hospital, sibling child care), these can be significant stressors for families. The absence of adequate healthcare insurance or Medicaid is presumed to be a risk factor for family stress. In a well-controlled study of 8- and 9-year-old children with spina bifida and their families, Holmbeck and colleagues (2002) found that socioeconomic status is associated with increased levels of family conflict and with an increase in stressful life events for both the families of children with spina bifida and families in the matched control group. However, socioeconomic status was a more potent predictor of family conflict for the families of children with spina bifida. Related findings were reported in another controlled study of high-risk, low-income youth with asthma, in which socioeconomic status combined with health risk status was highly predictive of psychological difficulties (Gillaspy, Hoff, Mullins, Van Pelt, & Chaney, 2002).

There is a well-established literature on the importance of social support and its role as a predictor of health outcome (House, Lanis, & Umberson, 1988), and specific evidence for its association with successful adaptation in childhood illnesses, including cancer and rheumatic disease (Hoeksta-Weebers, Jaspers, Kamps, & Klip, 2001; Kazak et al., 1995; Von Weiss et al., 2002). Although it has been long known that there are no differences in overall marital adjustment, separation, or divorce between families with and without children with medical disorders (Sabbeth & Leventhal, 1984), the presence of marital discord and other family problems is also a risk factor for ongoing difficulties.

The meaning that families make of the experience of having a child with healthcare needs may be related to later adjustment. Beliefs about illness have been explored primarily in the context of adult health (Rolland, 1994). The existing literature has been predominantly theoretical and clinical. However, looking at the related concept of family rituals in pediatric asthma, Markson and Fiese (2000) found that child anxiety was lessened in families with higher levels of commitment to family rituals, such as consistency in mealtime structure and types of foods, and to religious or social activities. Although this finding applies to families both with and without a child with asthma, it speaks to the importance of structure and meaning in reducing overall family stress and its potential impact on child health.

The additive impact of stressors, including changes for the better and for the worse, on adjustment is well established in both children (Goodyer, Kolvin, & Gatzanis, 1987) and adults (Kornblith et al., 2001). In the context of serious childhood illness, it is tempting to focus primarily on the child and the illness. This is necessary and important, but it is myopic if done in a way that excludes consideration of other stressors experienced by the child and family. Indeed, a social-ecological perspective argues for consideration of the many changes that unfold as the child grows and develops. The school setting is one in which there often is early recognition of the impact of non-illness-related family stressors or events (e.g., a child's parents separate; a family moves; there is a death in the family; a parent loses a job). The additive impact of these stressors for families of children with healthcare needs is similar to that of other families, although the potential to exceed the child's and family's capacity for coping effectively may be heightened when the additional stressors related to coping with illness are considered.

Collaborations among Families and Community Systems

Children and families bring unique mosaics of risk and competence to the challenges they face related to healthcare as it is provided across multiple settings. Although more focal in the cases of chronic pediatric illnesses, these processes are relevant to more routine and acute pediatric healthcare concerns as well. Understanding how families relate to community systems involved in the provision of health services and how these systems are connected with one another is critical to the design and evaluation of models of integrated care. There has been relatively little research related to these issues. From a social-ecological perspective, the interactions among families, healthcare settings, schools, and other community-based settings are best viewed as interactive and reciprocal (Kazak et al., in press). Ideally, the strengths and resources inherent in each setting complement one another, providing an integrated and responsive network of care.

Family-centered care (Johnson, 2000) affirms the prominent roles of families and community systems in pediatric healthcare. This model is widely accepted within children's hospitals, and its recommendations have led to the creation of consumer-oriented, family-focused services. In large part, family-centered care is likely successful because it acknowledges and strengthens relationships between families and service providers, and among healthcare providers. As another example, the Collaborative Family Healthcare Association (CFHA; *www.CFHA.org*) highlights the importance of involving family and community systems in the healthcare process (see Chapter 5 for a more extensive discussion). Although the family-centered movement has been rapidly gaining in prominence, healthcare centers vary greatly in their effectiveness in applying this model, and the consistency with which this model is implemented among families within the same institution or agency can vary dramatically.

A large body of literature has discussed the importance of family involvement in education to promote successful outcomes for children (see Christenson & Sheridan, 2001). Family involvement can assist the school in building its capacity to address the developmental needs of children, forming caring attachments with children, and providing services to children in a culturally relevant manner (Pianta & Walsh, 1996). A critical dimension of family involvement is reciprocal communication between parents and school professionals (Fantuzzo, Tighe, & Childs,

2000). Effective family–school communication can promote creative solutions to educational, social, and healthcare issues that arise among children and foster their development across systems. Dysfunctional family–school patterns may limit the exchange of useful information across systems, prevent the family and school from engaging in creative problem solving, and interfere with the development of strong teacher–child relationships (Power & Bartholomew, 1987). The presence of a health condition requiring frequent and meaningful communication between the family and school may serve to magnify the impact of a dysfunctional family–school relationship. Whereas healthy children who are coping adaptively in school may be minimally affected by a family–school relationship that is distant or strained, children with health problems, who are struggling to adapt in school, may be much more vulnerable to the impact of dysfunctional family–school patterns.

Another relationship that is critical to children with health conditions and their families is that between healthcare systems and the schools (Drotar, 1995). Children with health problems often need medical intervention during the course of the school day. For example, the treatment of asthma, ADHD, and diabetes typically involves the application of medical interventions during the school day, under the care of a physician from a primary care, clinic, or hospital setting. The school is an excellent source of information about the effectiveness of these interventions, as well as potential adverse side effects that can arise in their implementation (Power, Atkins, Osborne, & Blum, 1994). When the healthcare and school systems collaborate to exchange information about the effects and side effects of medical intervention, there is a greater likelihood that treatments can be effective. Unfortunately, these systems often are disconnected, requiring parents to serve in the role of linking the health and school systems, which is untenable for many families (Phelps, Brown, & Power, 2002).

Help-Seeking Patterns of Families

Families differ greatly in their patterns of health-seeking behavior. Some families are inclined to seek out proactively experts to address the health concerns they have about their child. They may utilize a variety of techniques (e.g., Internet searches, consultation with professionals) to investigate alternatives within and, at times, outside the geographic region in which they live to identify professionals whom they believe can help their child. Other families are oriented to seek the advice of primary care professionals when they have a health concern. Their decision about how to assist their child may depend heavily on the guidance of the primary care provider. Other families are inclined to seek the advice of community members, such as faith-based leaders, block captains, hair-dressers, neighbors, and extended family members, when they are concerned about a health issue, including a mental health concern (Freudenberg, 2000; Tucker, 2002).

Help-seeking patterns are determined by many factors, including the financial resources of families (Padgett, Patrick, Burns, Schlesinger, & Cohen, 1993). The type of insurance coverage a family has may limit direct access to experts or may require consultation with the primary care provider in determining whether an expert is needed. The financial resources of the family may determine whether it can afford an insurance option that permits a high degree of choice versus one that restricts access to specialists. Also, a family's financial resources may have a strong influence on the decision to incur expenses not covered by the family insurance plan.

Help-seeking patterns also may be determined by cultural factors that are influenced by racial and ethnic group membership. For example, McMiller and Weisz (1996) examined the initial help-seeking behaviors of families by interviewing them about their attempts to get assistance for mental health concerns prior to their first visit to a clinic. They found that African American and Hispanic/Latino families were much less likely than white families to seek out help from professionals or agencies before presenting to the clinic. For the minority families, most preclinic contacts were through informal networks, including families, neighborhood organizations, or faith-based organizations. In contrast, for white families, most of the preclinic contacts were through formal networks, including medical staff, mental health professionals, and school personnel.

Variations in help-seeking patterns may reflect culturally determined differences in thresholds for determining whether a set of behaviors is problematic. Caregivers from different cultural backgrounds have been found to differ in the extent to which they view a child's behavior as problematic and in need of professional assistance (Lambert et al., 1992). Caregiver concerns about being stigmatized by labels, or about being medicated or hospitalized may also influence the help-seeking patterns of families (Takeuchi, Bui, & Kim, 1993). These concerns may contribute to a mistrust of professionals, resulting in premature completion of treatment or nonadherence with intervention strategies (Sue, Fujino, & Takeuchi, 1991).

Assessing the Capacity of Systems: An Integrated Model

The help-seeking pattern of families is important for professionals to understand, because it strongly determines their preferred ways of accessing community-based services. The preferred system for families might be a primary care practice, the school, a neighborhood agency, or the extended family. As indicated, the capacity of the preferred service delivery system to address the health needs of the child and family depends upon the functional status of the child, the risk and resilience of the family, and the resources and collaborations existing among community-based systems. Figure 2.2 illustrates our model for how these dimensions intersect to determine whether community-based systems can adequately address the health needs of children.

According to our proposed model, the stronger the child's health status and developmental assets, the greater the resilience of the family, and the stronger the collaborations among community systems, the more likely the child will be able to function successfully in the community. In contrast, the greater the child's health and developmental needs, the greater the risk experienced by the family, and the weaker the collaborations among systems in the community, the less likely the child will be able to function successfully in the community. In cases in which the child's functioning is significantly compromised, and family and community resources are limited, frequent hospitalization and intensive follow-

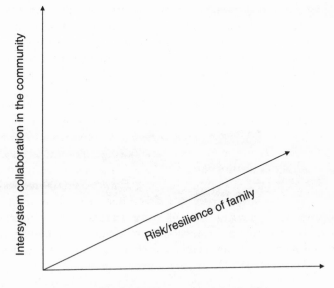

FIGURE 2.2. Factors that determine the capacity of a community-based system to effectively address the health needs of children.

up care in the community may be required to address the child's needs adequately. The following case description illustrates how these factors interact to determine how successfully the child is able to cope in the community.

Case Example

Jason, a 9-year-old third grader, attends public school in a middle-class, suburban neighborhood. Jason lives with his mother, Felicia, an Asian American single parent with three other children, ages 15, 11, and 7. Felicia has a general equivalency diploma (GED) and works approximately 50 hours a week, in two jobs. Health insurance for her children is provided through her primary employer and includes a fairly generous prescription plan and preventive medical care. Although she does not like her job, Felicia stays in it to receive a managed healthcare insurance plan that provides coverage for her children. She worries about how she would provide healthcare for her children if she changed jobs. Felicia often is fatigued but identifies as her major health concern her frequent use of cigarettes. During a recent episode of prolonged upper respiratory infection, the internist treating her suggested that she might be experiencing depression and suggested pharmacological treatment to see if the fatigue would remit. The doctor also discussed some lifestyle changes that might reduce the stress Felicia is experiencing and provided a referral for mental health counseling.

Felicia's mother lives with the family and works part-time as an administrative assistant at their church in the neighborhood. Felicia is divorced from Jason's father, Derrick. Derrick, an African American who lives with his second wife and young children in a nearby community, is also the father of Jason's 11-year-old brother, who has been diagnosed with ADHD. Derrick provides child support and maintains regular contact with his sons, including two or three visits a month.

Jason has had a history of moderate to severe asthma that was first identified when he was a toddler. Initially, Jason's asthma attacks were episodic, although some have been intense and frightening to Jason and his family, requiring urgent visits to the emergency room of the local hospital. Jason's healthcare is provided through a practice of six pediatricians. Although the practice advocates that each child have a primary pediatrician, Jason's visits are usually urgent, and he is seen by an available doctor or nurse practitioner. To prevent asthma attacks, Jason was prescribed cromolyn sodium, delivered via inhaler, four times per day. For the treatment of acute asthma attacks, a bronchodilator (albuterol), administered through an inhaler, has been prescribed (see Meyer & Blum, 1997, for a further description of these treatments).

Jason's performance in school is average academically. He is a quiet, somewhat withdrawn child, with two friends at school. School refusal has been a problem for Jason, even when he is free of asthma symptoms. According to the current teacher, the mother does not consistently encourage Jason to go to school. Felicia often seems to acquiesce to her son's demands to stay home with his grandmother or accompany her to work, where he can play and socialize with adults at the church.

A nurse is assigned to Jason's school 3 days a week. On the other days, a member of the school administrative staff has been authorized to attend to the children's health needs. Jason requires daily prophylactic treatment with cromolyn sodium at school and bronchodilator treatments as needed, which can be daily during periods in which his asthma attacks accelerate. Adherence to treatment in school and at home has been marginal. Felecia admits that she sometimes fails to administer the morning dose of cromolyn sodium because the household is hectic. Also, administration of the prophylactic medication in school has been inconsistent, particularly on days that the nurse is not available.

The relationship between the family and school is strained: Each party typically avoids the other (see Power & Bartholomew, 1987, for a description of an avoidant family–school relationship pattern). Jason's mother is upset that the school is not more consistent in the administration of the medication, and the school believes that Felicia reinforces school refusal by allowing Jason to miss school so often. School personnel also are frustrated to see that Felicia continues to smoke and feel that this is irresponsible behavior for a mother of a child with asthma. Jason has been treated in the emergency department of a nearby community hospital on four occasions over the past 6 months because of inability to manage asthma attacks. The pediatricians in the primary care practice express concern about the urgent visits to the emergency department and have provided Felicia with educational materials about asthma management. Felicia feels that they lecture her about it, and that they do not understand the pressures in her life.

This case illustrates how the child's health and developmental needs, the family's resources, and relationships among systems in the community interact to affect the capacity of the community to address this child's healthcare issues. Despite Jason's vulnerabilities (i.e., asthma, school refusal), he has a number of assets, including his adequate academic skills and strong relationships with two friends, that are valuable in enabling him to cope in the school and community. With regard to the family, Felicia is a single parent with healthcare issues of her own, but she is highly invested in the care of her children. Furthermore, the maternal grandmother and father appear to have strong relationships with the child. Although the health and school systems have a number of resources that can assist in addressing the child's health needs, linkages between these systems and the family are relatively weak. Jason and his family do not appear to have a strong relationship with a primary healthcare provider that could assist with medical management, including issues pertaining to nonadherence with asthma treatment and the mother's smoking in the home. A by-product of this underdeveloped collaboration is that Jason's asthma is treated symptomatically and reactively, often on an urgent basis in a hospital setting. Furthermore, the strained relationship between family and school precludes creative problem solving between these systems that could assist in the medical management of Jason during the school day and resolve concerns about school refusal. In addition, there is no evidence that the health and school systems are coordinated, which further contributes to problems addressing Jason's health and developmental needs.

What can be done to intervene in a situation like this? Major systems in Jason's life, family, school, and health system, are fractionated. The result is that Jason's health and emotional needs are not being addressed adequately, and his mother is left feeling isolated and overwhelmed in coping with his situation. Effective management requires an understanding of Jason's functioning within each system and an analysis of intersystem relationship patterns that promote and interfere with Jason's development. A critical concern is the identification of a professional who is able and willing to conduct an ecological assessment (see Chapter 3) and initiate an intervention plan that can strengthen relationships within and between these major systems, and orchestrate the actions of key stakeholders to provide coordinated care to Jason and his family.

Realistically, it may be most effective for the school to initiate change given the amount of time Jason spends in school each day and the resources of the school to address multiple domains of Jason's development, including the cognitive, social, emotional, and health domains. A school psychologist or psychologist linked with the school, for example, could assume the role of developing a framework for understanding linkages among systems, and collaborate with the family and professionals from various systems to develop an integrated service plan (see Kolbe et al., 1997, and Power, DuPaul, Shapiro, & Parrish, 1995, for a description of the roles school-based psychologists can serve in addressing the health needs of children).

CONCLUSIONS

Healthcare services increasingly are being provided in diverse settings, which is improving access to care and coordination of services, and contributing to a reduction in financial costs. The assets and limitations intrinsic to the major settings for the provision of healthcare (i.e., hospitals, primary care settings, schools, community-based agencies) provide a compelling justification for designing an integrated service delivery system that facilitates movement among these systems to capitalize on the assets of each. A critical feature of an effective service delivery system is that it be responsive to the needs and values of the families it is designed to serve. Families vary greatly in their inherent help-seeking patterns, and it is incumbent on the health system to be responsive to these tendencies. Numerous factors determine the extent to which a family's preferred method of seeking and receiving services can be effective in addressing the child's and family's health needs. These factors include (1) the medical condition and needs of the child, (2) the risk and resilience of the family, and (3) the level of integration among systems providing health services in the community. Understanding these factors can help to determine the appropriate setting for care at a particular point in time. Furthermore, an assessment of these variables can assist in identifying issues that need to be addressed in developing a comprehensive intervention plan for the child and family.

REFERENCES

American Academy of Pediatrics. (1996). *Diagnostic and statistical manual for primary care (DSM-PC), child and adolescent version.* Elk Grove Village, IL: Author.

Benson, P. L. (1997). *All kids are our kids: What communities must do to raise caring and responsible children and adolescents.* San Francisco: Jossey-Bass.

Best, M., Streisand, R., Catania, L., & Kazak, A. E. (2001). Parental distress during pediatric leukemia and posttraumatic stress symptoms (PTSS) after treatment ends. *Journal of Pediatric Psychology, 26,* 299–308.

Black, M., & Krishakumar, A. (1998). Children in low income urban settings: Interventions to promote mental health and well-being. *American Psychologist, 53,* 635–646.

Brown, K. J., & Roberts, M. C. (2000). Future issues in pediatric psychology: Delphic survey. *Journal of Clinical Psychology in Medical Settings, 7,* 5–15.

Brown, R. T. (Ed.). (1999). *Cognitive aspects of chronic illness in children.* New York: Guilford Press.

Brown, R. T., & Freeman, W. (2002). Primary care. In L. Marsh & M. Fristad (Eds.), *Handbook of serious emotional disturbance in children and adolescents* (pp. 428–444). New York: Wiley.

Christenson, S. L., & Sheridan, S. M. (2001). *Schools and families: Creating essential connections for learning.* New York: Guilford Press.

Comer, J. P., Haynes, N. M., Joyner, E. T., & Ben-Avie, M. (1996). *Rallying the whole village: The Comer process for reforming education.* New York: Teachers College Press.

Drotar, D. (1995). *Consulting with pediatricians: Psychological perspectives for research and practice.* New York: Plenum Press.

Drotar, D., & Zagorski, L. (2001). Providing psychological services in pediatric settings in an era of managed care: Challenges and opportunities. In J. N. Hughes, A. M. La Greca, & J. C. Conoley (Eds.), *Handbook of psychological services for children and adolescents* (pp. 89–104). New York: Oxford University Press.

Fantuzzo, J., Tighe, E., & Childs, S. (2000). Family Involvement Questionnaire: A multivariate assessment of family participation in early childhood education. *Journal of Educational Psychology, 92,* 367–376.

Freudenberg, N. (2000). Health promotion in the city: A review of current practice and future prospects in the United States. *Annual Review of Public Health, 21,* 473–503.

Gillaspy, S., Hoff, A., Mullins, L., Van Pelt, J., & Chaney, J. (2002). Psychological distress in high-risk youth with asthma. *Journal of Pediatric Psychology, 27,* 363–372.

Goodyer, I., Kolvin, I., & Gatzanis, S. (1987). The impact of recent undesirable life events on psychiatric disorders in childhood and adolescence. *British Journal of Psychiatry, 151,* 179–184.

Hoekstra-Weebers, J. E., Jaspers, J. P., Kamps, W., & Klip, E. C. (2001). Psychological adaptation and social support of parents of pediatric cancer patients: A prospective longitudinal study. *Journal of Pediatric Psychology, 26,* 225–236.

Holmbeck, G., Coakley, R., Hommeyer, J., Shapera, W., & Westhoven, V. (2002). Observed and perceived dyadic and systemic functioning in families of preadolescents with spina bifida. *Journal of Pediatric Psychology, 27,* 177–189.

House, J., Lanis, K., & Umberson, D. (1988). Social relationships and health. *Science, 241,* 540–545.

Institute of Medicine. (1994). *Reducing risks for mental disorders: Frontiers for preventive intervention research.* Washington, DC: National Academy Press.

Johnson, B. (2000). Family-centered care: Four decades of progress. *Families, Systems, and Health, 18,* 137–156.

Kazak, A., Barakat, L., Meeske, K., Christakis, D., Meadows, A., Casey, R., Penati, B., & Stuber, M. (1997). Posttraumatic stress, family functioning, and social support in survivors of childhood leukemia and their mothers and fathers. *Journal of Consulting and Clinical Psychology, 65,* 120–129.

Kazak, A. E., Rourke, M. T., & Crump, T. A. (in press). Families and other systems in pediatric psychology. In M. C. Roberts (Ed.), *Handbook of pediatric psychology* (3rd ed.). New York: Guilford Press.

Kazak, A. E., Segal-Andrews, A. M., & Johnson, K. (1995). Pediatric psychology research and practice: A family/systems approach. In M. C. Roberts (Ed.), *Handbook of pediatric psychology* (2nd ed., pp. 84–104). New York: Guilford Press.

Kazak, A. E., & Simms, S. (1996). Children with life-threatening illnesses: Psychological difficulties and interpersonal relationships. In F. Kaslow (Ed.), *Handbook of relational diagnosis and dysfunctional family patterns* (pp. 225–238). New York: Wiley.

Kazak, A., Stuber, M., Barakat, L., Meeske, K., Guthrie, D., & Meadows, A. (1998). Predicting postttraumatic stress symptoms in mothers and fathers of survivors of childhood cancer. *Journal of the American Academy of Child and Adolescent Psychiatry, 37*, 823–831.

Kids Count Data Online. (1999). Baltimore, MD: Annie E. Casey Foundation (*www.aecf.org*).

Kolbe, L. J., Collins, J., & Cortese, P. (1997). Building the capacity of schools to improve the health of the nation: A call for assistance from psychologists. *American Psychologist, 52*, 256–265.

Kornblith, A., Herndon, J., Zuckerman, E., Viscoli, C., Horwitz, R., Cooper, M., Harris, L., Tkaczuk, K., Perry, M., Budman, D., Norton, L., Hollan, J., & Cancer and Leukemia Group B. (2001). Social support as a buffer to the psychological impact of stressful life events in women with breast cancer. *Cancer, 91*(2), 443–454.

Kupst, M. J., Natta, M., Richardson, C., Schulman, J., Lavigne, J., & Das, L. (1995). Family coping with pediatric leukemia: Ten years after treatment. *Journal of Pediatric Psychology, 20*, 601–617.

Lambert, M. C., Weisz, J. R., Knight, F., Desrosiers, M., Overly, K., & Thesiger, C. (1992). Jamaican and American adult perspectives on child psychopathology: Further exploration of the threshold model. *Journal of Consulting and Clinical Psychology, 60*, 146–149.

Logan, D., Radcliffe, J., & Smith-Whitley, K. (2002). Parent factors and adolescent sickle cell disease: Associations with patterns of health service use. *Journal of Pediatric Psychology, 27*, 475–484.

Markson, S., & Fiese, B. (2000). Family rituals as a protective factor for children with asthma. *Journal of Pediatric Psychology, 25*, 471–479.

McMiller, W. P., & Weisz, J. R. (1996). Help-seeking preceding mental health clinic intake among African American, Latino, and Caucasian youths. *Journal of the American Academy of Child and Adolescent Psychiatry, 35*, 1086–1094.

Menaghan, E. (1999). Social stressors in childhood and adolescence. In A. V. Horwitz & T. L. Scheid (Eds.), *A handbook for the study of mental health: Social contexts, theories, and systems* (pp. 315–327). New York: Cambridge University Press.

Meyer, G. A., & Blum, N. J. (1997). Allergies and asthma. In G. G. Bear, K. M. Minke, & A. Thomas (Eds.), *Children's needs: II. Development, problems, and alternatives* (pp. 827–840). Bethesda, MD: National Association of School Psychologists.

National Center for Education in Maternal and Child Health. (2000). *Bright futures in practice: Mental health*. Washington, DC: Georgetown University Press.

Padgett, K., Patrick, C., Burns, B., Schlesinger, H., & Cohen, J. (1993). The effect of insurance benefit changes on use of child and adolescent outpatient mental health services. *Medical Care, 31*, 96–110.

Phelps, L., Brown, R. T., & Power, T. J. (2002). *Pediatric psychopharmacology: Combining medical and psychosocial interventions*. Washington, DC: American Psychological Association.

Pianta, R. C., & Walsh, D. (1996). *High-risk children in the schools: Creating tained relationships*. New York: Routledge.

Power, T. J., Atkins, M. S., Osborne, M. L., & Blum, N. J. (1994). The school chologist as manager of programming for ADHD. *School Psychology Review, 23*, 279–291.

Power, T. J., & Bartholomew, K. L. (1987). Family–school relationship patterns: An ecological assessment. *School Psychology Review, 14*, 222–229.

Power, T. J., & Blom-Hoffman, J. (in press). The school as venue for managing and preventing health problems: Opportunities and challenges. In R. T. Brown (Ed.), *The handbook of pediatric psychology in school settings*. Mahwah, NJ: Erlbaum.

Power, T. J., DuPaul, G. J., Shapiro, E. S., & Parrish, J. M. (1995). Pediatric school psychology: The emergence of a subspecialty. *School Psychology Review, 24*, 244–257.

Quittner, A., & DiGirolamo, A. (1998). Family adaptation to childhood disability and illness. In R. T. Ammerman & J. V. Campo (Eds.), *Handbook of pediatric psychology and psychiatry* (Vol. 2, pp. 70–80). Boston: Allyn & Bacon.

Roberts, M. C., & Hurley, L. K. (1997). *Managing managed care*. New York: Plenum Press.

Rolland, J. (1994). *Families, illness and disability: An integrative treatment model*. New York: Basic Books.

Sabbeth, B., & Leventhal, J. (1984). Marital adjustment to chronic childhood illness. *Pediatrics, 73*, 762–768.

Sameroff, A., Bartko, W., Baldwin, A., Baldwin, C., & Seifer, R. (1998). Family and social influences in the development of child competence. In M. Lewis & C. Feiring (Eds.), *Families, risk and competence* (pp. 165–185). Mahwah, NJ: Erlbaum.

Simms, S., & Kazak, A. E. (1998). Family systems interventions. In C. E. Coffey & R. A. Brumback (Eds.), *Textbook of pediatric neuropsychiatry* (pp. 1449–1464). Washington, DC: American Psychiatric Press.

Stancin, T., & Palermo, T. M. (1997). A review of behavioral screening practices in pediatric settings: Do they pass the test? *Journal of Developmental and Behavioral Pediatrics, 18*, 183–194.

Sue, S., Fujino, H., & Takeuchi, D. (1991). Community mental health services for ethnic minority groups: A test of the community responsiveness hypothesis. *Journal of Community and Clinical Psychology, 59*, 533–538.

Takeuchi, D., Bui, K., & Kim, L. (1993). The referral of minority adolescents to community mental health centers. *Journal of Health and Social Behavior, 34*, 153–164.

Tucker, C. M. (2002). Expanding pediatric psychology beyond hospital wall to meet the healthcare needs of ethnic minority children. *Journal of Pediatric Psychology, 27*, 315–324.

U.S. Department of Health and Human Services. (2001). *Mental health: Culture, race, and ethnicity: A supplement to mental health: A report of the Surgeon General*. Rockville, MD: U.S. Department of Health and Human Services, Substance Abuse and Mental Health Administration, Center for Mental

Health Services, National Institutes of Health, National Institute of Mental Health.

Vannatta, K., Gertstein, M., Short, A., & Noll, R. (1998). A controlled study of peer relationships of children surviving brain tumors. *Journal of Pediatric Psychology, 23*, 279–287.

Von Weiss, R., Rapoff, M., Varni, J., Lindsley, C., Olson, N., Madson, K., & Berstein, B. (2002). Daily hassles and social support as predictors of adjustment in children with pediatric rheumatic disease. *Journal of Pediatric Psychology, 27*, 155–165.

Wade, S. L., Borawski, E. A., Taylor, H. G., Drotar, D., Yeates, K. O., & Stancin, T. (2001). The relationship of caregiver coping to family outcomes during the initial year following pediatric traumatic injury. *Journal of Consulting and Clinical Psychology, 69*(3), 406–415.

Wade, S. L., Taylor, H. G., Drotar, D., Stancin, T., & Yeates, K. (1996). Childhood traumatic brain injury: Initial impact on the family. *Journal of Learning Disabilities, 29*, 652–661.

Wallander, J. L., Hubert, N. C., & Varni, J. W. (1988). Child and maternal temperament characteristics, goodness of fit and adjustment in handicapped children. *Journal of Clinical Psychology, 17*, 366–344.

PART II

Developing
Intervention Strategies

CHAPTER 3

Designing Interventions

Integrating Assessment Paradigms

Reliable and valid assessment data must be collected prior to, during, and after treatment implementation to ensure that interventions are comprehensive and effective. In particular, decisions regarding intervention targets, as well as where, when, and how to intervene, are optimized when based on information regarding child, family, and school functioning. Over the years, several assessment and evaluation paradigms have been proposed to promote understanding and effective treatment for childhood disorders (Mash & Terdal, 1997). The major assessment models include (1) diagnostic/categorical, (2) dimensional or empirical, (3) functional, and (4) ecological paradigms. Each model has unique strengths and limitations, particularly regarding information provided to support effective treatment design.

4models

The purpose of this chapter is to provide an overview of each of the four assessment models, with a particular emphasis on their relative advantages and disadvantages for the evaluation of children with physical and/or mental disorders. Because no single assessment paradigm provides sufficient information about child functioning, we discuss how data can be integrated across models such that one model's strengths counterbalance another's weaknesses. After data are gathered and integrated, one must be able to link the results of an assessment to treatment design and implementation. This linkage is discussed with a specific focus on functional assessment data. Once an intervention plan has been put into place, data continue to be gathered to document whether the intervention has been implemented as intended and whether desired outcomes have been obtained. Thus, we delineate how information collected within each of the four paradigms can contribute to intervention

51

evaluation and ongoing modifications to treatment. Next, the use of these assessment models in home, school, and community settings is explicated by discussing practical issues and potential limitations. Finally, we present two cases to illustrate how assessment data are interpreted and integrated to design interventions for children with physical or mental disorders.

DESCRIPTION OF ASSESSMENT PARADIGMS

Several paradigms have been developed to facilitate the assessment of children's needs and to plan potentially effective intervention strategies. Each paradigm is based upon a unique set of assumptions and espouses the use of specific strategies to guide the assessment of child functioning. The following is a description of four paradigms that are commonly used in research and practice and have been demonstrated to be highly useful in understanding children's needs.

Categorical Assessment

Categorical assessment typically is used to determine whether an individual meets criteria for a particular diagnosis. This paradigm has been developed primarily within the field of medicine, but it has made a strong contribution to research and practice in other fields, including psychology. The criteria for making this decision generally are derived by a panel of experts after a thorough review of the research literature pertaining to the diagnostic condition. The criteria may be further shaped by field testing of provisional criteria to evaluate the ability of each proposed symptom to differentiate children known to have the disorder from those known not to have the disorder (e.g., see Frick et al., 1994). In addition, field testing can be useful in identifying the number of symptoms needed to optimize the prediction of clinically meaningful levels of impairment (e.g., see Lahey et al., 1994).

The fourth edition of the *Diagnostic and Statistical Manual of Mental Disorders* (DSM-IV; American Psychiatric Association, 1994) is a categorical system widely used in the United States for determining whether individuals meet criteria for one or more mental health disorders (e.g., posttraumatic stress disorder, conduct disorder, autistic disorder). Clinicians make determinations about whether a diagnosis is present or absent based on criteria specified in this manual, which were derived by a panel of experts, primarily psychiatrists.

Diagnostic interviews commonly are used to assist clinicians in making categorical decisions about the presence or absence of mental health disorders. Interview procedures can vary with regard to their level of structure, but most are highly systematic and provide specific guidelines for requesting information and following up with probes. Diagnostic interviews differ with regard to their scope. Some interview techniques, such as the Autism Diagnostic Interview—Revised (Lord, Rutter, & LeCouteur, 1994), assess a narrow range of diagnostic entities. However, most diagnostic interviews examine a broad range of categories. Examples of some of the commonly used broadband, structured interviews are the Diagnostic Interview System for Children (DISC; Shaffer et al., 1996), the Diagnostic Interview for Children and Adolescents (DICA; Reich, Leacock, & Shanfeld, 1995), and the Kiddie–Schedule of Affective Disorders—Present and Lifetime Version (K-SADS-PL; Kaufman, Birmaher, Brent, Rao, & Ryan, 1996). Many structured interviews have been adapted for administration to parents as well as children.

The psychometric properties of diagnostic interviews vary greatly depending on the informant and the disorder being assessed. For children under the age of 14 years, the reliability and validity of interviews generally are more favorable when the informant is a parent as opposed to a child. Furthermore, parent-reported interviews generally are more psychometrically sound for externalizing as opposed to internalizing disorders (Schwab-Stone et al., 1996).

Categorical methods of assessment have some notable strengths. These methods can provide a framework for assessment by delineating the domains and specific symptoms that need to be evaluated. Categorical procedures help clinicians to organize clinical information, relate clinical findings to known and often validated patterns of behavior, explore potential correlates associated with diagnostic patterns, and predict developmental outcomes (Power & Eiraldi, 2000). Identifying the presence of a disorder can alert the clinician to a risk for serious functional impairment and can be useful in identifying potentially useful pharmacological and psychosocial treatments (see Phelps, Brown, & Power, 2002).

Categorical methods are also associated with several limitations. These methods identify the child as the source of the problem and fail to provide information about systemic factors that contribute to a child's difficulties (Power & DuPaul, 1996). Identifying merely the presence or absence of disorder does not account for gradations of symptom severity. Children may have subclinical levels of symptomatology, yet still encounter some level of impairment. Addressing the needs of these children was one of the main reasons the *Diagnostic and Statistical Manual for Primary Care—Child and Adolescent Version* (American Academy of Pediatrics, 1996) was created (Drotar, 1999). Of great concern is that categorical methods do not account for important differences in symptom presentation and severity across gender and developmental levels. Furthermore, categorical methods provide only limited information about how to design psychosocial and educational interventions (Gresham & Gansle, 1992).

Dimensional Assessment

The dimensional approach provides an assessment of domains related to various aspects of physical, cognitive, behavioral, emotional, and social functioning. These methods assess functioning along a continuum generally ranging from adaptive to nonadaptive, with no clear demarcation of the boundary between disordered and nondisordered (Achenbach & McConaughy, 1996). These approaches typically provide an assessment of the severity of functioning related to each dimension by comparing the child's level of functioning to that of peers of similar gender and age. Historically, the dimensions assessed using these methods have been derived empirically from parent, teacher, and self-ratings of behavior (Achenbach & McConaughy, 1996), although more recently, the dimensions are being derived on the basis of empirical as well as rational methods (Achenbach & Rescorla, 2001; Reynolds & Kamphaus, 1992).

Behavior rating scales frequently are used to provide a dimensional assessment of functioning. Rating scales can be differentiated with regard to their scope of assessment. Some rating scales are multiaxial and assess multiple domains of behavioral, emotional, social, and academic functioning. Examples of these types of measures, often referred to as broadband scales, are the Child Behavior Checklist (CBCL; Achenbach & Rescorla, 2001), the Behavior Assessment System for Children (BASC; Reynolds & Kamphaus, 1992), and the Devereux Scales of Mental Disorders (DSMD; Naglieri, LeBuffe, & Pfeiffer, 1994). Rating scales also have been developed to assess a narrow range of functioning. The number of narrowband constructs that have been assessed using rating scales is virtually limitless. Just a few examples of these measures are the ADHD Rating Scale-IV (DuPaul, Power, Anastopoulos, & Reid, 1998), the Social Skills Rating System (SSRS; Gresham & Elliott, 1990), and the Multidimensional Anxiety Scale for Children (March, 1997).

Behavior rating scales also differ with regard to the informant providing clinical information. Some rating scales have been developed for use with multiple informants, including the parent, teacher, and child (e.g., CBCL, BASC, SSRS). Also, procedures have been designed to assess peer-oriented social functioning through peer ratings (Asher & Dodge, 1986).

The psychometric properties of rating scales generally are strong. The construct validity of these measures often is supported through exploratory and confirmatory factor analyses. The reliability of the multiple subscales of these measures typically is demonstrated through indices of internal consistency and test–retest reliability. Furthermore, research regarding the association of these scales with measures of related constructs and the lack of association of these measures with scales of different constructs often is available to support the convergent and divergent validity of the instruments.

Because dimensional methods of assessment generally are norm-referenced, they are highly useful for determining the severity of symptom clusters. These approaches can provide information about how children function in real-life settings from multiple informants. Furthermore, rating scales can assess functioning across settings, in particular the home and school. Limitations of these approaches include their susceptibility to rater bias. Informants may vary greatly in the thresholds they apply in making determinations about whether a behavior is problematic (Reid & Maag, 1994). Also, rating scales typically are developed for use with the general population of children, and they may not be responsive to racial, ethnic, or cultural differences among children (Reid et al., 1998). Furthermore, dimensional approaches have limited treatment utility. These methods are helpful in understanding the range and severity of children's problems across settings, but they provide little information about the meaning and function of behavior, which can be highly useful in intervention design.

Functional Assessment

A number of terms have been used to describe functional assessment procedures (e.g., descriptive analysis, functional analysis, and functional behavioral assessment). In addition, problem-solving models of assessment (see Ikeda et al., 2002; Sheridan, Kratochwill, & Bergan, 1996) typically recommend the use of functional methods of assessment. The use of these various terms has led to some confusion as to what the term functional assessment actually means (see Haynes & O'Brien, 1990). For our purposes in this chapter, functional assessment refers to a *broad* set of procedures that examine the environmental events that maintain target behaviors (Horner, 1994). More specifically, functional assessment includes procedures that comprise a descriptive analysis (e.g., interviews, and direct observations of target behaviors and environmental events as they naturally occur), as well as those strategies used in an experimental analysis (e.g., systematic *manipulation* of environmental events to examine the functional relationship between the target behaviors and environmental events).

The goal of functional assessment is identifying environmental contingencies that maintain target behaviors (e.g., escape from anxiety-provoking medical procedures) as well as establishing operations (e.g., fatigue due to lack of sleep) and/or antecedent events (e.g., presentation of an academic task) that may set the occasion for target behaviors to occur. Information gathered during the functional assessment can be used to determine which interventions are most likely to be effective for a specific child within a specific setting. In fact, a rich literature base in the fields of developmental disabilities (Iwata et al., 1994) and behavior disorders (Kern, Childs, Dunlap, Clarke, & Falk, 1994) documents the efficacy of interventions designed using functional assessment data.

A comprehensive functional assessment includes three steps: (1) interviewing, (2) descriptive analysis, and (3) experimental analysis (for details of these steps, see Nelson, Roberts, & Smith, 1998). In most applied circumstances, a functional assessment involves interviews and the collection of descriptive data rather than direct manipulation of environmental contingencies by the assessor (see Nelson et al., 1998, for discussion of this issue). Although one cannot incontrovertibly determine function through a descriptive assessment, by conducting interviews with a variety of sources (e.g., student, parent, teacher, nursing staff) and observing the target behaviors in relation to environmental events, the topography of the behavior can be defined, and a potential function for the target behavior can be hypothesized (Nelson et al., 1998). Interventions can then incorporate the hypothesized function to change behavior in the desired direction. For example, if a student is hypothesized to engage in off-task behavior to gain peer attention (i.e., commonly referred to as "class clown" behavior), then the intervention should include attention from peers contingent on appropriate, on-task behavior (e.g., peer tutoring) (for more examples, see DuPaul & Ervin, 1996).

Functional assessment procedures have several positive features. Chief among these is that specific intervention strategies can be derived directly from these data (i.e., minimal inference is required). If the data support a specific behavioral function in a certain setting, then one can design an intervention for the setting that addresses behavioral function in a relatively straightforward manner. Another strength of functional assessment is that it involves examining behavior in a natural context. Child behavior is seen as inextricably linked to environmental events that precede and follow it. In addition, child behavior itself serves as an antecedent and/or consequent event for the behaviors of peers and adults in the same setting. Finally, functional assessment is based on the premise that individuals differ with respect to why they engage in specific behaviors despite the fact that they may share certain attributes (e.g., diagnosis, gender, and ethnicity). Stated differently, functional assessment goes beyond a search for a generic linkage between a diagnosis and a treatment, wherein the richness of individual differences is acknowledged.

Several factors can limit the utility of functional assessment (DuPaul, Eckert, & McGoey, 1997). First, there are practical constraints associated with this methodology, including the time and effort involved in collecting data, as well as the degree to which the parent, teacher, or healthcare provider is involved in the assessment process. A second potential limitation is that experimental analysis procedures may actually increase problematic behavior, albeit temporarily. It is important to consider whether the "cost" associated with conducting an assessment that temporarily increases inappropriate behavior is justified if an effective intervention can be determined in a more efficient manner, thereby reducing long-term "costs" associated with the inappropriate behavior that is already exhibited by the student. This limitation is yet another reason why practitioners prefer to use descriptive rather than experimental analysis procedures in applied settings. Another limitation is that functional assessment procedures have been designed principally for the treatment of externalizing problems, and they may have less utility for addressing emotional issues. Furthermore, functional assessment does not provide information relevant to diagnostic decisions or to predicting outcomes based on diagnostic status. A final potential problem with functional assessment methods is that, in some instances, the data will not clearly delineate the function of the problematic behavior. It also is possible for one behavior to have multiple functions and for interventions to have limited applicability to other settings. In such instances, the psychologist must decide whether to design an intervention that addresses one or both hypothesized functions, and whether separate interventions are needed across relevant settings. Intervention decisions typically are based on clinical judgment that takes into account practical constraints, cost-efficiency, and relative likelihood of success among intervention alternatives.

Ecological Assessment

Developmental–ecological theory (Bronfenbrenner, 1979) provides a conceptual foundation and useful framework for designing ecological methods of assessment. Ecological methods are intended for the assessment of an individual's functioning within systems as well as dimensions of systems that have been shown to have an impact on the developing person. The hallmark of ecological assessment is an examination of the contexts in which individuals function, with a particular emphasis on relationships among individuals within systems. Although, historically, these methods, like most approaches to assessment, have emphasized the examination of deficits, more recently, the focus has increasingly been placed on identifying competencies and contextual assets (e.g., Epstein & Sharma, 1998; Fantuzzo, Tighe, & Childs, 2000).

Rating scales commonly are used to assess dimensions of systems and relationships among individuals in systems. One of the most widely used measures of the family system is the Parenting Stress Index (PSI; Abidin, 1995), a parent report scale that provides an assessment of two domains of parenting stress: The Child Domain reflects stress related to characteristics of the child (i.e., Adaptability, Acceptability, Demandingness, Mood, Distractibility/Hyperactivity, and Reinforces Parent), and the Parent Domain reflects stress related to characteristics of the parent (i.e., Depression, Attachment to Child, Role Restriction, Competence, Isolation, Spousal Relationship, and Health). Family measures have been developed that focus more directly on assessing the parent–child relationship. To cite examples, the Conflict Behavior Questionnaire (Robin & Foster, 1989), and the Parent–Child Relationship Questionnaire (Furman & Giverson, 1995) are measures of parent–child interaction based on both parent and child report. Measures of marital functioning, such as the Dyadic Adjustment Scale (Spanier, 1976), also have been used commonly in research and clinical practice.

Numerous procedures have been developed to assess dimensions of the school system. The Index of Teaching Stress (Greene, Abidin, & Kmetz, 1997), which is similar in structure to the PSI, provides an assessment of both child and teacher factors that contribute to teacher stress. The Student–Teacher Relationship Scale (Pianta, 2002) assesses teachers' feelings and beliefs about their interactions with children. In addition, several measures of school climate have been designed to assess important dimensions of the school ecology that have been demonstrated to have an effect on learning and social development. For example, the School Climate Survey (Haynes, Emmons, Ben-Avie, & Comer, 1996) is designed to assess numerous dimensions of school environment through the collection of informant reports from students, parents, and teachers. In addition, direct observation procedures, such as the Code for Instructional Structure and Student Academic Response (CISSAR; Stanley & Greenwood, 1981), have been developed to assess classroom variables related to engagement in academic work.

Ecological methods also have been used to understand relationships between systems. For example, the Family Involvement Questionnaire (Fantuzzo et al., 2000) and the Parent–Teacher Involvement Questionnaire (Kohl, Lengua, & Robert, 2000) have been developed to assess parental involvement in education at home and school, as well as the quality of parent–teacher communications.

Unlike other assessment paradigms, the ecological approach provides information about contextual factors impacting child functioning and critical relationships in a child's life. These data can be highly useful in identifying contextual dimensions that need to be targeted for intervention. A limitation is that many of these procedures are still in the preliminary stages of development. Although these methods tap dimensions that are critical for the comprehensive understanding of child functioning, the results may need to be interpreted with caution when used in clinical practice. Given the challenges of assessing variables targeted in ecological assessment (i.e., relational dynamics), it is understandable that the psychometric properties of these types of methods generally are poorer than dimensional methods that assess more discreet aspects of behavior. Scale development of ecological measures is certainly a fruitful area for investigation in the future.

INTEGRATING ASSESSMENT DATA ACROSS PARADIGMS

As indicated in the previous section, many assessment paradigms potentially are useful in understanding children's developmental needs. Each of these paradigms is associated with numerous strengths and limitations, which are summarized in Table 3.1. In examining this table, it is worth noting that the limitations of one paradigm are often the strengths of another paradigm. For example, categorical methods can help to organize clinical information about a child and provide valuable information about potential risk factors, but these strategies focus solely on the child, emphasize deficits, and fail to account for important contextual factors that influence behavior. In contrast, ecological methods provide invaluable information about important contextual variables, and identify assets of the child and context that can promote healthy development. However, ecological strategies generally provide more limited information about the child. Likewise, dimensional methods yield useful information about the range and severity of child problems but are limited in their utility for treatment planning. In contrast, functional methods generally are useful in generating hypotheses about the meaning and purpose of behavior that can be helpful for treatment planning. However, functional methods may focus on a narrow range of concerns and typically are more useful in addressing externalizing than internalizing problems.

A comparison of the strengths and limitations inherent in these paradigms strongly suggests that they can be thought of as complementary

TABLE 3.1. Comparing Alternative Assessment Paradigms

Paradigm	Strengths	Limitations
Categorical	Provides a framework for assessment. Identifies potential risk factors. Useful in predicting developmental outcomes. Identifies potentially useful interventions.	Identifies child as source of problem. Fails to identify gradations in symptom severity. Fails to account for gender and age differences. Limited utility in planning psychosocial interventions.
Dimensional	Useful in assessing problem severity. Accounts for gender and age differences. Useful in conducting multi-informant assessment. Measures generally are psychometrically sound.	Subject to informant bias. May not be responsive to cultural differences. Fails to assess contextual variables. Limited utility of planning psychosocial interventions.
Functional	Assesses purpose of behavior. Accounts for contextual influences. Focuses on building skills and reducing deficits. Useful in developing psychosocial interventions.	Limited for assessing pathology and predicting outcomes. Can have adverse effects in the short run. Limited utility in assessing internalizing symptoms. Can be time consuming.
Ecological	Provides an assessment of contextual variables. Assesses the status of critical relationships. Focuses on assessing assets as well as deficits. Useful in identifying resources for intervention.	Limited for understanding child psychological variables. Limited for understanding function of behavior. Based on limited normative data. Generally based on limited psychometric data.

in many ways. The implication is that an approach to assessment and intervention planning that includes multiple and perhaps all of these paradigms often is the most advantageous. Later in this chapter, we describe two case studies that incorporate each of these paradigms in conducting a comprehensive assessment of a child's needs and in designing a potentially effective intervention plan.

LINKING ASSESSMENT TO INTERVENTION

Assessment data traditionally have been used to delineate problematic areas and to make diagnostic decisions. Ultimately, however, these data are most useful when they can pinpoint possible treatment directions and guide the design of specific intervention plans, in part, through identification of individual, family, and systemic strengths. For this reason, assessment measures should not only have adequate psychometric properties (i.e., reliability and validity) but also should have demonstrated treatment utility (Kratochwill & McGivern, 1996). Categorical assessment leading to diagnosis can aid in treatment selection to the extent that a research literature is available linking specific treatments to specific diagnoses. For example, a variety of studies have demonstrated the effectiveness of behavioral parent training for children with oppositional defiant disorder (e.g., Brestan & Eyberg, 1998). In similar fashion, dimensional assessment measures are helpful in determining broad areas of functioning that may be problematic (i.e., potential treatment targets), as well as those areas of strength that can be capitalized upon in a treatment plan. Furthermore, dimensional data can highlight the severity of problematic behaviors and therefore help to determine how intensive intervention procedures need to be. For instance, children with more severe levels of ADHD symptoms may require the combination of stimulant medication and behavior modification rather than relying solely on the latter (Barkley, 1998). Information derived from ecological assessment measures provides a broader, systemic view that aids in treatment planning. Specifically, ecological data may aid in determining the (1) environments where treatment is needed; (2) potential impact of treatment on family, school, and community systems; (3) individuals who can be useful in implementing interventions; and (4) areas in which possible unintended effects (i.e., side effects) may occur.

When it comes to deciding on specific intervention components, functional assessment data are critical, particularly when designing treatment plans that include behavioral strategies. In fact, we have found it useful to conceptualize functional assessment as the endpoint of an assessment funnel that directly links assessment data to intervention design (see Figure 3.1). From a treatment-planning perspective, categorical and dimensional data provide broad directions for intervention selection. Ecological assessment data contribute more specific information about environmental and systemic factors that need to be addressed in intervention design. At the most specific level of analysis, functional assessment data indicate which interventions are most likely to be effective in which environments by indicating the possible function of the target behavior.

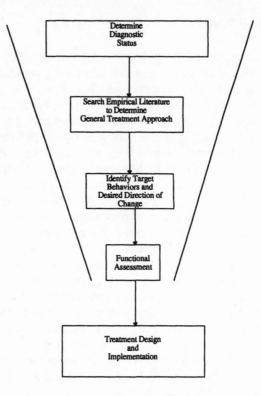

FIGURE 3.1. Funnel of assessment procedures for designing interventions for children with behavioral difficulties. From DuPaul and Ervin (1996). Copyright 1996 by the Association for Advancement of Behavior Therapy. Reprinted by permission.

Once the function of a child's behavior is determined, then an intervention is designed that leads to functionally equivalent behavior. Functionally equivalent interventions provide access to desired consequences contingent on appropriate rather than problematic behavior. Connections between behavioral functions, and possible functionally equivalent interventions, are displayed in Figure 3.2. For example, if a child engages in disruptive behavior in a classroom to gain teacher attention, then the intervention should arrange for teacher attention to be contingent only on the display of appropriate behavior, while disruptive behavior is ignored (i.e., differential reinforcement of incompatible behavior). It is assumed that function-based interventions will be more effective than strategies implemented based on broader diagnostic data and/or a trial-and-error approach. Furthermore, because function-based interven-

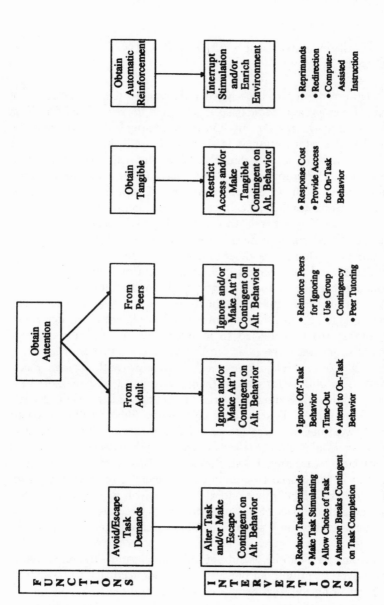

FIGURE 3.2. Possible functions for child behavior and associated interventions. From DuPaul and Ervin (1996). Copyright 1996 by the Association for Advancement of Behavior Therapy. Reprinted by permission.

tions provide access to desired consequences, it is presumed that these strategies will result in outcomes that are maintained over time.

MONITORING OUTCOMES AND ONGOING ASSESSMENT

Once an intervention plan is designed and implemented, the collection of assessment data on a periodic basis is suggested for several reasons. First and foremost, gathering information from a variety of sources helps to ensure that the intervention is leading to desired outcomes (i.e., that goals are being met). Second, data regarding treatment outcomes and integrity of implementation can be used to make informed decisions about ongoing modifications to the treatment plan. Detailed feedback can be given to parents, teachers, healthcare professionals, and the students themselves regarding what is working and what aspects of treatment need to be altered. Finally, the social validity of outcomes for target students can be evaluated to determine whether performance has been "normalized" and the degree to which interventions are viewed as acceptable and feasible by those charged with implementation.

As part of the treatment planning process, the treatment team (including parents and healthcare professionals) collaborate to determine what data are to be collected to monitor outcomes. Ideally, psychometrically sound measures that are directly related to treatment goals will be used. For example, if one is seeking to improve the academic performance of a child with cancer, then curriculum-based measurement probes in math and reading (i.e., brief "tests" of academic skills derived directly from the child's classroom curriculum; Shinn, 1998) could be collected two times per week to assess acquisition of skills over time. Areas of functioning closely related to treatment targets and/or assumed to be affected by treatment also should be assessed. If, for instance, a medication is being used to alter a child's behavior (e.g., methylphenidate for treating ADHD), behavioral outcomes will be of primary interest; however, the impact of this treatment on related areas, such as academic achievement and social functioning should be assessed (see Chapter 6).

Outcome data can be useful not only to determine the relative success of the intervention plan but also to provide feedback to those who are implementing the treatment (e.g., parents and teachers). To the extent that certain treatment components are working, these will be retained, while other, less successful components may need to be modified, discarded, and/or replaced. Feedback to treatment agents is further enhanced through collection of intervention integrity data. Integrity can be assessed through direct observation of the treatment being implemented (by someone other than the treatment agent, or through review of audio-tapes or videotapes of treatment sessions), self-report of completed treatment steps (by the treatment agent), and/or direct examination of products generated by treatment (e.g., self-monitoring checklists completed the student). These data can help determine the degree to which the overall plan is being implemented accurately, which treatment components are being inaccurately implemented, and where training efforts may be needed (see Chapter 9 regarding evaluation of prevention programs for more details).

Although it is important to document clinically significant changes in targeted performance areas, it is equally critical to assess whether obtained changes are considered socially valid by treatment "consumers" (e.g., parents, teachers, and children). Social validity can be assessed in at least two ways. First, one can document the degree to which performance is "normalized" (i.e., similar to selected peers). For example, behavioral observation data can be collected for both the target student and typical peers in the same environment. A second way to evaluate social validity is by obtaining consumer satisfaction ratings from parents, teachers, and children. Consumers can provide their perceptions regarding the relative success, feasibility, and satisfaction of the intervention, as well as the degree to which they would use the specific treatment strategies in the future.

PRACTICAL CHALLENGES AND ISSUES

Although the assessment model proposed in this chapter has many advantages for use in evaluating children, a number of factors present challenges for implementation in applied settings. Chief among these factors are the limitations associated with finite resources including money, time, lack of training of key personnel, and/or the lack of available personnel. A comprehensive assessment clearly can exhaust resources even under the best of conditions. Thus, practitioners may have to select assessment procedures that balance informational needs and limited resources. Alternatively, one might advocate for changes at the system level to free up additional resources (e.g., by arguing that more resources over the short term may save money over the long term by preventing more costly difficulties from arising) or seek funding from external sources (e.g., foundation or Federal grants).

Another challenge to implementation of a comprehensive assessment model is the feasibility of using certain assessment procedures (e.g., functional analyses) in "real-world" settings. Although functional analyses involving the direct manipulation of contingent events are critical to determining definitively the function of challenging behavior, these are difficult to conduct in classroom, healthcare, and home settings. First, the manipulation of some consequent events (e.g., peer attention) following problematic behavior may prove unwieldy and/or be seen as unacceptable by teachers and parents. Second, the fact that the target behavior will be increased, at least temporarily, by functional analyses can make the latter very difficult to "sell" to administrators, teachers, and parents. Finally, unless teachers or parents are trained to conduct functional analyses themselves, these procedures can be costly in terms of professional time and effort. For these reasons, functional assessments conducted in home, school, and healthcare settings typically include only descriptive assessment methods, which are less time-intensive and more acceptable to key stakeholders.

A third challenge to a comprehensive assessment model is the natural variability of child behavior across development. Changes in child functioning associated with different settings and caretakers, and the developmental maturation process results in assessment data that are time- and context-sensitive. Thus, periodic reassessments are necessary to ensure that a child's functioning is accounted for at the present time and under current circumstances. For example, the function of a child's disruptive behavior in math class could vary from school year to school year depending on situational factors and other variables.

CASE ILLUSTRATIONS

To illustrate the integration of assessment data across paradigms, two case descriptions are presented. The first case involves the evaluation of potential psychological and educational difficulties in a child being treated for cancer. A second case delineates the assessment of an elementary-school-age child exhibiting high levels of noncompliance and rule-breaking behavior at home and school.

Pediatric Cancer

Jennifer, a 15-year-old, Caucasian adolescent, was diagnosed with acute lymphocytic leukemia (ALL) at the age of 14. Jennifer lives with her father, an executive at a local technology company, and mother, a nurse who does not currently work outside the home but is active in several community organizations. Jennifer's father has had drinking problems in the past. Jennifer has one older brother, John, a first-year student at an Ivy league university on an athletic scholarship, and a younger sister,

Emily, age 10. Jennifer attends a public high school, where she takes honors courses and is active in several clubs. She maintains excellent grades and is considered to be talented in multiple academic skills areas. Although it has been difficult to maintain her athletic activities at her prediagnosis level, she is a strong tennis player and remains on the basketball team. In general, people have always described Jennifer as a "worrier" and very conscientious. Although she has typically been close with her parents, in the past couple of years, she has more conflicts with them about her autonomy.

Jennifer was a healthy child who rarely needed to see a doctor. During a visit to the emergency room at her local hospital for a fall during basketball practice, the doctor asked about multiple recent bruises. Subsequent to a blood test, Jennifer's parents were advised to have her evaluated immediately by a pediatric oncologist at the tertiary care center. On the 2-hour trip to the hospital, Jennifer became agitated and was unable to calm herself. Once at the hospital, a bone marrow aspiration was performed. Unfortunately, Jennifer, who was not well sedated during the procedure, remained very agitated while a large needle was inserted in her back for the procedure, and she recalls the pain vividly to this day. Her parents felt helpless in the situation. Jennifer was emotionally distraught when told that she had cancer and expressed anxiety that she would die.

The early months of chemotherapy were extremely difficult for Jennifer. (For a description of treatment approaches for ALL and their potential side effects, see Armstrong, Blumberg, & Toledano, 1999.) She became withdrawn, very anxious prior to each chemotherapy administration, and fearful of having her friends see her as her hair fell out and her weight increased (as a chemotherapy side effect). In addition to having nausea from the chemotherapy, she developed anticipatory nausea and vomiting on the way to the hospital for each weekly treatment. When her parents, siblings, friends, or teachers asked about her treatment, she refused to answer their questions. She also avoided another student at her school who had cancer and refused to watch television shows about medical issues. Her teachers and classmates responded favorably to a school reintegration program, and the principal offered flexibility in terms of attendance and opportunities for breaks during the day. Her oncologist asked one of the cancer center's psychologists to consult with the school team. Their questions related to her overall emotional well-being, and acute and chronic anxiety/distress.

Jennifer's case is not unusual for an adolescent girl with little prior experience coping with illness. She is a highly competent adolescent who has struggled to maintain her family, academic, athletic, and social lives as much as possible. A year into treatment, she is doing better than she appeared at diagnosis, although still having some difficulties. This is not unusual, but rather typical of the course of improvement seen over the first year subsequent to a diagnosis of a serious pediatric illness (Kazak, Rourke, & Crump, in press). In examining this situation, it is clear that Jennifer displayed symptoms of anxiety and depression at the time of diagnosis and for some time afterwards. From a categorical perspective, it is reasonable to assess whether she meets criteria for a depressive or anxiety disorder. Similarly, one year after her diagnosis, and given her symptoms of avoidance, it is reasonable to explore whether she may meet criteria for a diagnosis of posttraumatic stress disorder (PTSD).

Although it is possible that Jennifer could meet criteria for a DSM-IV disorder, it is more probable that her symptoms are at a subclinical level. Nonetheless, her anxiety, depressive, and posttraumatic stress symptoms arouse concern and contribute to functional impairments. Use of dimensional approaches of assessment by administering rating scales to the parents, teachers, and to Jennifer herself can be highly useful in determining the extent of her internalizing difficulties.

In the course of consulting with Jennifer, her parents, and the treatment team about her acute distress during medical procedures, a functional analysis can be helpful. It is reasonable to hypothesize that Jennifer's anticipatory nausea and vomiting are conditioned responses; that is, her initial administration of chemotherapy resulted in severe nausea that was subsequently paired with environmental cues. Her distress before and during procedures can be understood by examining the parameters of the procedures and the interactions among Jennifer, her parents, and the treatment team prior to, during and after treatment. For example, there may be ways in which Jennifer's parents could respond to help her calm herself. Indeed, highly effective relaxation and cognitive-behavioral interventions that interrupt learned patterns of behavior (e.g., anxiety in response to the treatment center) and teach new ways of responding are readily available (Powers, 1999).

Jennifer also can be understood within the context of her family and other systems. Using an assessment measure of family psychosocial risk and resilience in pediatric oncology (i.e., Psychosocial Assessment Tool; Kazak et al., 2001), the strengths of this family, including the presence of two involved parents, financial resources, and helpful connections with neighbors, community, and school, could be identified. Questions about the father's drinking and Jennifer's tendency toward internalizing symptoms are issues that could increase the overall psychosocial risk of the family. The relationship between Jennifer and her parents needs to be explored further, because communication problems may be preventing the parents from being as supportive as they would like to be. One of the primary treatment goals is to help the family to remain organized in a manner that promotes ongoing development for all members of the family.

Noncompliant Behavior

Brady, a 10-year-old Caucasian boy, attends fourth grade in a general education classroom in a suburban elementary school. He lives with his parents and younger sister, Keri (age 6), and his socioeconomic background can be characterized as middle class. Although his teacher reports that Brady is on grade level in most academic areas, problems have arisen regarding the degree to which he complies with teacher directives, completes his work, and follows school rules. Brady's parents also report a great deal of difficulty getting him to follow through on household chores and homework, as well as problems getting along with his younger sister. Furthermore, he reportedly defies their directives on a regular basis. Brady has several friends at school and in the neighborhood, although incidents involving verbal and physical aggression with other boys have increased in frequency over the past several months.

As a result of these concerns, Brady's parents have brought him to a clinical psychologist in their community for a psychological evaluation. Multiple assessment methods incorporating several respondents were used to gain an understanding of Brady's behavior difficulties in the context of home and school settings. Measures included diagnostic interviews with Brady, as well as his parents and teacher (by telephone), behavior rating scales completed by his parents and teacher, a self-report questionnaire completed by Brady, observations of parent–child interactions in several clinic-based analog situations, and collection of archival data (e.g., report cards) and permanent products (e.g., completed class work) from school.

Information gleaned from the diagnostic interviews provided data that were helpful from a categorical perspective. Specifically, Brady's parents and teacher reported significant symptoms of oppositional defiant disorder (ODD) as well as some symptoms of both attention-deficit/hyperactivity disorder (ADHD) and conduct disorder, although his behavior did not meet DSM-IV (American Psychiatric Association, 1994) criteria for either of the latter two disorders. Corroborating a diagnosis of ODD, parent and teacher ratings on the CBCL (Achenbach & Rescorla, 2001) indicated clinically significant elevations (i.e., T score > 70) on the Aggression and Social Problems subscales. Furthermore, he received borderline significant ratings (i.e., T score > 65) on the Attention Problems and Conduct Problems scales. Thus, from a dimensional point of view, Brady is reported to display problems with defiance, noncompliance, and verbal aggression to a greater degree than 98% of similar-age boys across home and school settings. Interestingly, Brady did not report significant problems in any area in the context of the diagnostic interview or on the Youth Self-Report Version of the CBCL (Achenbach & Rescorla, 2001). This is not surprising; children with externalizing behavior disorders are not necessarily reliable reporters of their symptoms (McMahon & Estes, 1997). Brady's problematic behaviors have led to a deterioration in his school performance; his report cards and other school archival data indicate a decline from "A" to "C" level performance (relative to previous school years) and more frequent disciplinary actions (e.g., being sent to the principal's office following incidents of verbal aggression).

Brady and his mother were observed while interacting in several clinic analog situations. These situations included Brady being asked to play alone while his mother completed a questionnaire, Brady and his mother being asked to complete a jigsaw puzzle together, and Brady being asked to complete several tasks (e.g., cleaning up the playroom) by his mother. An observer located behind a one-way mirror coded the percentage of intervals when Brady exhibited either noncompliant, verbally and physically aggressive behavior, as well as the percentage of intervals when Brady's mother showed either positive or negative attention toward him. The results of this observation indicated that Brady exhibited noncompliant and verbally aggressive behavior primarily during the task condition. Furthermore, his mother responded to his noncompliance by reprimanding him and threatening further disciplinary action (e.g., restricting his home activities). Although a formal experimental analysis was not conducted, observational data may be helpful in hypothesizing the function of Brady's noncompliant behavior. Specifically, it seems that parent-directed tasks are antecedent events that trigger Brady's verbal aggression and defiance. Furthermore, his noncompliant behavior appears to allow him to avoid, at least temporarily, tasks that are aversive.

Brady's parents and teacher also completed several questionnaires (e.g., PSI, Index of Teacher Stress) to examine the impact of his behavior in the context of home and school systems. Although his parents and teacher reported clinically significant levels of stress in interacting with Brady around task situations, they also reported him to have notable strengths, including cognitive and athletic abilities. Furthermore, his parents and teacher appeared to be highly motivated to work with Brady and believed that they had support from extended family members and school administrators.

The results of this assessment were used to design an intervention plan for home and school to reduce the frequency of Brady's noncompliant behavior, while promoting positive interactions with adult authority figures. Because his defiant behavior appears to be motivated by a desire to avoid effortful work, several options for presenting tasks were included in the plan. First, efforts to assign tasks that are interesting to Brady were encouraged, so that assignments would be seen as less aversive to him. Second, a choice-making strategy was designed wherein Brady would be given several options for completing an assignment (e.g., choose one of three math assignments). This provided Brady with some control, albeit limited, over the task situation. Finally, the time parameters for tasks were adjusted, wherein Brady would be provided with brief "attention breaks" following the completion of a subset of an assignment. For example, his parents would allow him to take a 5-minute break following completion of 25% of his homework. In addition to changing the ways that tasks were presented to him, a contingency management plan was implemented, wherein Brady gained access to preferred activities contingent on timely and quiet completion of assigned tasks. Included in these preferred activities were opportunities to interact with his parents (e.g., playing catch with his father) in an enjoyable context, in order to promote better relations among family members.

CONCLUSIONS

Comprehensive evaluation of child functioning requires an integrative model that incorporates categorical, dimensional, functional, and ecological assessment methods. Although each of the four assessment paradigms has specific limitations, each offers unique information that is critical to understanding a child and his or her familial and school context. Furthermore, assessment does not end with diagnosis but, rather, is an ongoing process, wherein data are collected to design and evaluate intervention strategies. Despite the challenges posed by limitations encountered in applied settings, comprehensive evaluation incorporating reliable and valid assessment methods is vital to understanding children with health disorders.

REFERENCES

Abidin, R. R. (1995). *Parenting Stress Index* (3rd ed.). Lutz, FL: Psychological Assessment Resources.

Achenbach, T. M., & McConaughy, S. H. (1996). Relations between DSM-IV and empirically-based assessment. *School Psychology Review, 25,* 329–341.

Achenbach, T. M., & Rescorla, L. A. (2001). *Manual for the ASEBA School-Age Forms and Profiles.* Burlington, VT: University of Vermont, Research Center for Children, Youth, and Families.

American Academy of Pediatrics. (1996). *Diagnostic and statistical manual for primary care—child and adolescent version.* Elk Grove Village, IL: Author.

American Psychiatric Association. (1994). *Diagnostic and statistical manual of mental disorders* (4th ed.). Washington, DC: Author.

Armstrong, F. D., Blumberg, M. J., & Toledano, S. R. (1999). Neurobehavioral issues in childhood cancer. *School Psychology Review, 28,* 194–203.

Asher, S. R., & Dodge, K. A. (1986). Identifying children who are rejected by their peers. *Developmental Psychology, 22,* 444–449.

Barkley, R. A. (1998). *Attention-deficit hyperactivity disorder: A handbook for diagnosis and treatment* (2nd ed.). New York: Guilford Press.

Brestan, E. V., & Eyberg, S. M. (1998). Effective psychosocial treatments of conduct-disordered children and adolescents: 29 years, 82 studies, and 5,272 kids. *Journal of Clinical Child Psychology, 27,* 180–189.

Bronfenbrenner, U. (1979). *The ecology of human development.* Cambridge, MA: Harvard University Press.

Drotar, D. (1999). The Diagnostic and Statistical Manual for Primary Care (DSM-PC), Child and Adolescent Version: What pediatric psychologists need to know. *Journal of Pediatric Psychology, 24,* 369–380.

DuPaul, G. J., Eckert, T. L., & McGoey, K. E. (1997). Interventions for students with attention deficit hyperactivity disorder: One size does not fit all. *School Psychology Review, 26,* 369–381.

DuPaul, G. J., & Ervin, R. A. (1996). Functional assessment of behaviors related to attention-deficit/hyperactivity disorder: Linking assessment to intervention design. *Behavior Therapy, 27,* 601–622.

DuPaul, G. J., Power, T. J., Anastopoulos, A. D., & Reid, R. (1998). *ADHD Rating Scale–IV: Checklists, norms, and clinical interpretation.* New York: Guilford Press.

Epstein, M. H., & Sharma, J. M. (1998). *Behavioral and Emotional Rating Scale: A strength-based approach to assessment.* Austin, TX: Pro-Ed.

Fantuzzo, J., Tighe, E., & Childs, S. (2000). Family Involvement Questionnaire: A multivariate assessment of family participation in early childhood education. *Journal of Educational Psychology, 92,* 367–376.

Frick, P. J., Lahey, B. B., Applegate, B., Kerdyck, L., Ollendick, T., Hynd, G. W., Garfinkel, B., Greenhill, L., Biederman, J., Barkley, R. A., McBurnett, K., Newcorn, J., & Waldman, I. (1994). DSM-IV field trials for the disruptive behavior disorders: Symptom utility estimates. *Journal of the American Academy of Child and Adolescent Psychiatry, 33,* 529–539.

Furman, W., & Giverson, R. (1995). Identifying the links between parents and their children's sibling relationships. In S. Shulman (Ed.), *Close relationships and socioemotional development* (pp. 95–108). Norwood, NJ: Ablex.

Greene, R. W., Abidin, R. R., & Kmetz, C. (1997). The Index of Teaching Stress: A measure of student–teacher compatibility. *Journal of School Psychology, 35,* 239–260.

Gresham, F. M., & Elliott, S. N. (1990). *Manual for the Social Skills Rating System—Parent, teacher, and self-report forms.* Circle Pines, MN: American Guidance Service.

Gresham, F. M., & Gansle, K. A. (1992). Misguided assumptions of DSM-III-R:

Implications for school psychological practice. *School Psychology Quarterly,* 7, 79–95.

Haynes, N. M., Emmons, C., Ben-Avie, M., & Comer, J. P. (1996). *The school development program: Student, staff and parent–school climate surveys.* New Haven, CT: Yale Child Study Center.

Haynes, S. N., & O'Brien, W. H. (1990). Functional analysis in behavior therapy. *Clinical Psychology Review, 10,* 649–668.

Horner, R. H. (1994). Functional assessment: Contributions and future directions. *Journal of Applied Behavior Analysis, 27,* 401–404.

Ikeda, M. J., Grimes, J., Tilly, W. D., Allison, R., Kurns, S., & Stumme, J. (2002). Implementing an intervention-based approach to service delivery: A case example. In M. R. Shinn, H. M. Walker, & G. Stoner (Eds.), *Interventions for academic and behavior problems: II. Preventive and remedial approaches.* Bethesda, MD: National Association of School Psychologists Publications.

Iwata, B. A., Pace, G. M., Dorsey, M. F., Zarcone, J. R., Vollmer, T. R., Smith, R. G., Rodgers, T. A., Lerman, D. C., Shore, B. A., Mazaleski, J. L., Goh, H. L., Cowdery, G. E., Kalsher, M. J., McCosh, K. C., & Willis, K. D. (1994). The functions of self-injurious behavior: An experimental–epidemiological analysis. *Journal of Applied Behavior Analysis, 27,* 215–240.

Kaufman, J., Birmaher, B., Brent, D., Rao, U., & Ryan, N. (1996). *Kiddie-Schedule of Affective Disorders—Present and Lifetime Version.* Pittsburgh, PA: Western Psychiatric Institute and Clinic.

Kazak, A., Prusak, A., McSherry, M., Simms S., Beele, D., Rourke, M., Alderfer, M., & Lange, B. (2001). The Psychosocial Assessment Tool (PAT): Development of a brief screening instrument for identifying high-risk families in pediatric oncology. *Families, Systems and Health, 19,* 303–317.

Kazak, A. E., Rourke, M. T., & Crump, T. A. (in press). Families and other systems in pediatric psychology. In M. C. Roberts (Ed.), *Handbook of pediatric psychology* (3rd ed.). New York: Guilford Press.

Kern, L., Childs, K. E., Dunlap, G., Clarke, S., & Falk, G. D. (1994). Using assessment-based curricular intervention to improve the classroom behavior of a student with emotional and behavioral challenges. *Journal of Applied Behavior Analysis, 27,* 7–20.

Kohl, G. O., Lengua, L. J., & Robert, J. (2000). Parent involvement in school: Conceptualizing multiple dimensions and their relations with family and demographic risk factors. *Journal of School Psychology, 38,* 501–523.

Kratochwill, T. R., & McGivern, J. E. (1996). Clinical diagnosis, behavioral assessment, and functional analysis: Examining the connection between assessment and intervention. *School Psychology Review, 25,* 342–355.

Lahey, B. B., Applegate, B., McBurnett, K., Biederman, J., Greenhill, L., Hynd, G. W., Barkley, R. A., Newcorn, J., Jensen, P., Richters, J., Garfinkel, B., Kerdyk, L., Frick, P. J., Ollendick, T., Perez, D., Hart, E. L., Waldman, I., & Shaffer, D. (1994). DSM-IV field trial for attention-deficit hyperactivity disorder in children and adolescents. *American Journal of Psychiatry, 151,* 1673–1685.

Lord, C., Rutter, M., & LeCouteur, A. (1994). Autism Diagnostic Interview—Revised: A revision of the diagnostic interview for caregivers of individuals with possible pervasive developmental disorders. *Journal of Autism and Developmental Disorders, 24, 659–685.*

March, J. S. (1997). *Multidimensional anxiety scale for children (MASC).* North Tonawanda, NY: Multi-Health Systems.

Mash, E. J., & Terdal, L. G. (Eds.). (1997). *Assessment of childhood disorders* (3rd ed.). New York: Guilford Press.

McMahon, R. J., & Estes, A. M. (1997). Conduct problems. In E. J. Mash & L. G. Terdal (Eds.), *Assessment of childhood disorders* (3rd ed., pp. 130–193). New York: Guilford Press.

Naglieri, J. A., LeBuffe, P. A., & Pfeiffer, S. I. (1994). *Manual for the Devereux Scales of Mental Disorders.* San Antonio, TX: Psychological Corporation.

Nelson, J. R., Roberts, M. L., & Smith, D. J. (1998). *A practical guide for conducting functional behavioral assessments in school settings.* Longmont, CO: Sopris-West.

Phelps, L., Brown, R. T., & Power, T. J. (2002). *Pediatric psychopharmacology: Combining medical and psychosocial interventions.* Washington, DC: American Psychological Association.

Pianta, R. C. (2002). *Student–Teacher Relationship Scale.* Odessa, FL: Psychological Assessment Resources.

Power, T. J., & DuPaul, G. J. (1996). Attention-deficit/hyperactivity disorder: The re-emergence of subtypes. *School Psychology Review, 25,* 284–296.

Power, T. J., & Eiraldi, R. B. (2000). Educational and psychiatric classification systems. In E. S. Shapiro & T. R. Kratochwill (Eds.), *Behavioral assessment in schools (2nd ed., pp. 464–488). New York: Guilford Press.*

Powers, S. (1999). Empirically supported treatments in pediatric psychology: Procedure-related pain. *Journal of Pediatric Psychology, 24,* 131–145.

Reich, W., Leacock, N., & Shanfeld, K. (1995). *Diagnostic Interview for Children and Adolescents—parent version.* St. Louis, MO: Washington University, Division of Child Psychiatry.

Reid, R., & Maag, J. W. (1994). How many fidgets in a pretty much: A critique of behavior rating scales for identifying students with ADHD. *Journal of School Psychology, 32,* 339–354.

Reid, R., DuPaul, G. J., Power, T. J., Anastopoulos, A. D., Rogers-Atkinson, D., Noll, M. B., & Riccio, C. (1998). Assessing culturally different students for attention deficit hyperactivity disorder using behavior rating scales. *Journal of Abnormal Child Psychology, 26,* 187–198.

Reynolds, C.R., & Kamphaus, R. W. (1992). *Manual for the Behavior Assessment System for Children.* Circle Pines, MN: American Guidance Service.

Robin, A. L., & Foster, S. L. (1989). *Negotiating parent–adolescent conflict: A behavioral–family systems approach.* New York: Guilford Press.

Schwab-Stone, M. E., Shaffer, D., Dulcan, M. K., Jensen, P. S., Fisher, P., Bird, H. R., Goodman, S. H., Lahey, B. B., Lichtman, J. H., Canino, G., Rubio-Stipec, M., & Rae, D. S. (1996). Criterion validity of the NIMH Diagnostic Interview Schedule for Children Version 2.3 (DISC-2.3). *Journal of the American Academy of Child and Adolescent Psychiatry, 35,* 878–888.

Shaffer, D., Fisher, P., Dulcan, M. K., Davies, M., Piacentini, J., Schwab-Stone, M. E., Lahey, B. B., Bourdon, K., Jensen, P. S., Bird, H. R., Canino, G., & Regier,

D. A. (1996). The NIMH Diagnostic Interview Schedule for Children Version 2.3 (DISC-2.3): Description, acceptability, prevalence rates, and performance in the MECA study. *Journal of the American Academy of Child and Adolescent Psychiatry, 35,* 865–877.

Sheridan, S. M., Kratochwill, T. R., & Bergan, J. R. (1996). *Conjoint behavioral consultation: A procedural manual.* New York: Plenum Press.

Shinn, M. R. (Ed.). (1998). *Advanced applications of curriculum-based measurement.* New York: Guilford Press.

Spanier, G. B. (1976). Measuring dyadic adjustment: New scales for assessing the quality of marriage and similar dyads. *Journal of Marriage and Family, 38,* 15–28.

Stanley, S. D., & Greenwood, C. R. (1981). *Code for instructional structure and student academic response: Observer's manual.* Kansas City: Juniper Gardens Children's Project, Bureau of Child Research, University of Kansas.

CHAPTER 4

Integrating Children with Health Problems into School

In response to reforms in healthcare and education, there has been increased emphasis on addressing the needs of children with medical conditions in community and school settings. Among the many changes occurring in the healthcare system, the managed care movement has precluded the hospitalization of many children with serious health needs and has resulted in a briefer duration of hospitalization for many who are admitted (Roberts & Hurley, 1997). As a result, there has been increasing reliance on community-based resources, including the school, to address the needs of children with serious medical conditions. The emphasis in healthcare reform on increasing the accessibility and coordination of services for children and families has also affirmed the critical role of the school as a venue for delivering healthcare services (Carlson, Tharinger, Bricklin, DeMers, & Paavola, 1996; Holtzman, 1992; Short & Talley, 1997).

Changes in educational law have highlighted the responsibility of the school in addressing the needs of children with special health conditions. Under the provisions of the Individuals with Disabilities Education Act (IDEA; 1997), children with acute and chronic health conditions whose educational performance is substantially affected by their illnesses may be eligible for services and protections afforded in the special education system. Even if children with health conditions do not require special education, they may be eligible for safeguards provided by Section 504 of the Rehabilitation Act of 1973 (Riccio & Hughes, 2001). Educational law has emphasized that children with disabilities, including those with medical conditions, are entitled to receive services in the least restrictive and most normalized setting feasible given the nature and extent of their impairments.

This chapter reviews the school problems that children with health conditions may encounter and the challenges that families, peers, and school personnel often face in addressing these children's needs. School programs developed to address the concerns of children with special health needs are critically reviewed. In this chapter, we propose a model of school integration based on principles of social-ecological theory and behavioral consultation. The model emphasizes the importance of linking the healthcare, educational, and family systems to resolve problems and promote competence among children with health conditions. A case is described to illustrate the steps of school integration.

THE CHALLENGE OF SCHOOL

Children with health conditions often experience significant challenges adapting to school. Those with disabilities or chronic illnesses that arise in early childhood (e.g., autism, Down syndrome, asthma, and pediatric HIV) may face challenges with school integration from the beginning of elementary school. Others may acquire an illness or disorder that interrupts developmentally appropriate functioning (e.g., cancer, traumatic brain injury [TBI], and muscular dystrophy), resulting in significant, acute problems with school reintegration.

Factors Contributing to School Problems

The school challenges encountered by children with health problems vary as a function of numerous factors (Sexon & Madan-Swain, 1993). The nature of the child's medical condition obviously is an important factor, and children with the same illness can differ greatly in the challenges they experience in school (see Phelps, 1998). The problems children encounter in school can vary as the course of the condition unfolds. For example, with TBI, a child's neuropsychological functioning can change dramatically during the first several months after the trauma (Clark, Russman, & Orme, 1999). Also, the developmental level of the child is usually a critical factor. For example, the emotional and social concerns that an adolescent with cancer experiences are typically very different from those of an elementary-school-age child (Worchel-Prevatt et al., 1998).

The child's experience in school may be related to the beneficial and adverse effects of the medical treatments being used. For example, medications for seizure disorders may vary in their effectiveness from child to child and may be associated with adverse effects on attention and memory (Black & Hynd, 1995). The child's and family's adherence with intervention, which may be strongly influenced by the quality of the collaboration between the family and health professionals (see Chapter 5), may determine the extent to which treatment is effective. In addition, the school ecology, the teacher's knowledge and skills in working with the child, and the relationship between family and school can have an impact on the child's school experience (Worchel-Prevatt et al., 1998).

Effects on School Performance

Medical conditions can have an effect on children's school performance in many ways. Some health conditions, such as cancer and asthma, may result in heightened levels of school absenteeism, which is often associated with poor academic performance and a sense of social isolation (Weitzman, 1986). Many health conditions, particularly those that involve the central nervous system, have an effect on the child's cognitive functioning, which in turn can have a deleterious effect on academic achievement (see Brown, 1995). Furthermore, although children with chronic illnesses have been shown to be remarkably resilient with regard to their peer functioning (Vannatta, Gertstein, Short, & Noll, 1998) and psychological adjustment (Kazak, 2001), they often experience significant coping challenges within the family, school, and peer group (see Kazak, Rourke, & Crump, in press).

Health problems can have an effect on significant persons in a child's life, which in turn can have an impact on school functioning. Teachers may be uncertain about how to instruct a child with health problems. They often have concerns about how to address the behavioral, emotional, and social problems these children present in school (Chekryn, Deegan, & Reid, 1987), which could have an effect on the quality of the teacher–child and family–school relationships. Peers may not know how to relate to a child with health problems and may engage in behavior that is neglectful or rejecting of the child (Prevatt, Heffer, & Lowe, 2000). Furthermore, parents may have ambivalent feelings about sending their ill child to school, and they may lack confidence in the teacher's ability to work effectively with their child (Sexon & Madan-Swain, 1993).

PROGRAMS TO FACILITATE SCHOOL INTEGRATION

Most of the research related to school integration has focused on the school reentry of children with cancer and TBI. Children with a wide range of other disabilities and illnesses also may experience significant problems with school integration and reintegration. Nonetheless, models of programming for children with cancer and TBI may be applicable for children with these other conditions. The following is a brief review of the types of programs that have been described in the literature.

Skills Building Programs

One approach to intervention has been to focus on enhancing the strategies and skills of the child with the illness. There are numerous examples of programs that have been established to build individual skills and strategies for children with disabilities and illnesses. Cognitive remediation, which is often applied with children who have TBI or a brain tumor, is designed to improve the child's cognitive assets and to develop compensatory strategies in areas of cognitive weakness (Mateer, Kerns, & Eso, 1997). Social skills training, which has been applied with children who have a broad range of disabilities and illnesses, is designed to facilitate the development of children's skills in social perception, problem solving, and emotion regulation (Farmer & Peterson, 1995). Research regarding the effectiveness of programs focused on developing individual skills has been very limited. At this point, there is little empirical support for these methods, although clinicians often report that they have a high level of utility. Likewise, concerns have been raised about the effectiveness of these types of interventions in improving academic and social performance in actual school settings over extended periods of time (Clark et al., 1999; DuPaul & Eckert, 1994).

Teacher Education Programs

The purpose of teacher education initiatives is to (1) provide instruction to teachers about a particular medical condition, (2) describe attitudes that children and their families may have about the condition, (3) describe the challenges that children with this condition often experience in school, and (4) present strategies for assisting children in the areas of academic, social, and emotional functioning (Prevatt et al., 2000). Workshops often are presented by one or more health professionals, including physicians, nurses, pediatric psychologists, and social workers. These programs typically improve teacher knowledge about a specific illness and teacher perceptions of self-efficacy in addressing the needs of children with health conditions (e.g., see Ross, 1984). Unfortunately, data regarding the effectiveness of these programs in improving child outcomes typically are lacking (Prevatt et al., 2000).

Peer Education Programs

Peer education initiatives typically are designed to improve the level of peer support offered to children with disabilities and illnesses in school.

During these programs, peers receive instruction about (1) the potential impact of illness on children, (2) the unique challenges of children with illnesses, (3) the difficulties these children may experience with peer interactions, and (4) strategies for providing peer support. A variety of strategies, including verbal instruction, modeling, and role playing, often are used to facilitate the educational process. Research has demonstrated that these programs frequently lead to improvements in peer knowledge about medical conditions and increased interest in interacting with children who are ill (e.g., see Benner & Marlow, 1991). Alternatively, research has not clearly demonstrated that these programs have a beneficial effect on peer behavior in interactions with ill children (Treiber, Schramm, & Mabe, 1986). Furthermore, these programs often fail to consider potentially adverse effects on children with illnesses and disabilities (Prevatt et al., 2000), such as social isolation from peers or self-consciousness on the part of the child with a medical condition.

Multicomponent Programs

The most successful school integration programs typically include multiple intervention components and make provisions for extended follow-up care. A critical component is understanding and facilitating the child's adjustment in the family system (Farmer & Peterson, 1995; Worchel-Prevatt et al., 1998). The presence of an illness or disability can have a significant effect on parent–child and sibling relationships (Kazak & Simms, 1996). Clinicians can serve a critical role in assessing relationship patterns that emerge in response to illness and in facilitating family interaction patterns that promote healthy development. A family that is able to adapt successfully to illness can be invaluable in assisting with the child's adjustment to school by engaging teachers in collaborative problem solving, and by supporting educational activities (e.g., homework, parent tutoring, and educational computer games) in the home environment (see Christenson & Sheridan, 2001).

Another essential component is the orientation of personnel in the school system (Katz, Varni, Rubenstein, Blew, & Hubert, 1992). Sharing information about the child's illness through written materials and brief presentations can be useful in preparing educators. In addition, teachers need information about the specific needs of the child with an illness and consultation about intervention strategies. For example, teachers may need to develop strategies to address frequent absences from school, problems in acquiring academic skills, deficits in attention and self-control, and problems with peer interaction. In many cases, children need an individualized education plan through IDEA or an individualized service plan through Section 504. Clinicians can be highly useful in promoting collaborative relationships among the family, school professionals, and healthcare providers to develop potentially effective, socially valid, and feasible intervention plans (Clark et al., 1999).

Addressing the child's needs for support in peer interactions also is an important intervention component (Katz et al., 1992). Educating peers about the child's illness and working with them to develop strategies to assist the child in peer interactions may be useful in promoting successful school integration. However, many children with chronic health conditions require more intensive intervention that may involve social skills training for target children, the inclusion of nontarget peers in the intervention program, and training of school personnel to prompt and reinforce the use of effective social strategies (Glang, Todis, Cooley, Wells, & Voss, 1997).

Because the school status of a child with a medical condition can vary markedly over time, particularly in the early stages of illness, the inclusion of a follow-up component is necessary (Katz et al., 1992). School personnel, health professionals, and families can benefit from ongoing consultation to monitor the child's progress and modify the educational plan as needed.

SCHOOL INTEGRATION MODEL

Regardless of the type of intervention program that one uses to facilitate the integration of children with health problems into the school setting, success depends on the effectiveness of the process through which the program is delivered, as well as the specific strategies employed. The concept of integration referred to here is the full participation of students with health problems into the fabric of everyday life within the school setting. The literature regarding integration has been focused primarily on students with health problems who have been physically removed from the school setting because of a medical concern and are reintroduced into the schools (see Prevatt et al., 2000). Our view of the integration process, which is similar to the concept of inclusion in special education (Individuals with Disabilities Education Act, 1997), is broader and includes those students with health concerns who have been excluded from many of the daily activities (e.g., recess and physical education class) of the school setting. Although they are not physically removed from the school building, they may be psychologically excluded from ongoing school life, resulting in poor attachment with teachers and a sense of isolation from peers (Worchel-Prevatt et al., 1998).

Given that families of children with health problems receive advice from numerous professionals about strategies for school integration, establishing strong connections between educational and medical professionals is essential. Linking professionals from different systems can be a challenge, considering the differences in models of service delivery (e.g., medical vs. functional model), domains of care (e.g., medical, mental health, and educational), vocabulary specific to each discipline, and the methods used to evaluate outcomes. An additional challenge to successful collaboration is that professionals from various disciplines and systems need to communicate a clear, unified set of messages to families in order to promote successful school integration. The process of establishing and maintaining strong connections among the family, healthcare, and school systems is as important as the specific strategies used to assist the child with integration.

Developmental–ecological theory (Bronfenbrenner, 1979) provides a highly useful framework for establishing a process to link the family, healthcare, and school systems to facilitate school integration. According to Bronfenbrenner's model, it is essential to know how a child functions within each major system in which he or she operates, and to understand how functioning in each system serves to promote or impede adaptation in another system (Pianta, 2001). Understanding child adaptation within and across multiple contexts requires multi-informant, multimethod assessment involving the input of family members, school personnel, and healthcare professionals.

Linking assessment with intervention in the process of integration can be facilitated by an understanding of the functional relationships between child behavior and the biopsychosocial contexts in which the child operates. Although template approaches to treatment that involve the matching of intervention protocols to individual symptoms or symptom clusters may have some clinical value, treatment generally is more effective when strategies are tailored to address the unique functional relationships that exist between behavior and biopsychosocial determinants (DuPaul & Ervin, 1996; Kratochwill & McGivern, 1996). The field of applied behavior analysis includes a set of methods that have been demonstrated to be highly useful in understanding these functional relationships and in devising individualized intervention plans.

Furthermore, the process of integration must be continuous with modification of the intervention based on data collected through a formative evaluation process. The monitoring of student progress must be responsive to the needs of the child as well as the changing capacity of the family, school, and healthcare systems to meet these needs.

Figure 4.1 illustrates a model for integrating students with health problems into the schools. The model involves a two-phase process that is implemented in four steps. The first three steps, occurring at the preintegration phase, focus on enabling the child with a medical condition to function competently within the family system and establishing a foundation for the family and school to collaborate effectively with each other. The fourth step (i.e., the integration stage) encompasses the actual process of school integration, as well as efforts to maintain successful school–family–healthcare system partnerships over time.

Although the first three steps may unfold in a sequential pattern, it is preferable that they occur simultaneously. The key focus of the preintegration phase is to strengthen the family and school systems, and to build connections between them, so that the foundations of successful integration programs exist before the actual intervention is implemented. Without this preliminary work, any form of consultation, including the model used in the fourth step, is likely to fail. The following is a description of each step.

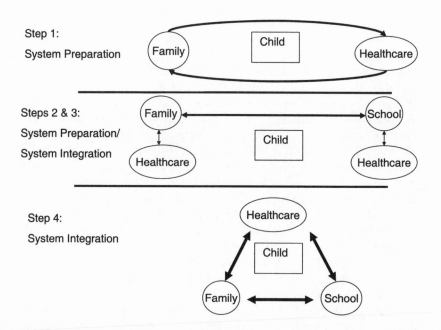

FIGURE 4.1. Steps involved in the integration of children with health problems into school. In Step 1, the healthcare team partners with the family to address the child's medical condition. In Steps 2 and 3, the healthcare team collaborates with family members to prepare them for collaboration with the school and establishes a partnership with school team members to prepare them for collaboration with the family. In Step 4, the healthcare team, school team, and family are involved in a conjoint health promotion and problem-solving process.

Preintegration: Step 1. Strengthening the Family

Coping with medical conditions involves many unique challenges that can be highly stressful for children and their parents (Kazak, Segal-Andrews, & Johnson, 1995). Although research has affirmed that families of children with chronic health conditions generally are highly resilient (Holmbeck, Coakley, Hommeyer, Shapera, & Westhoven, 2002; Kazak et al., in press), families vary widely in their adaptation to illness. Characteristics of the illness, the child, and family appear to moderate the vulnerability of families to the stressors presented by a chronic illness (Wallander & Thompson, 1995). For example, illnesses that are potentially life threatening and those that have significant effects on neurocognitive functioning are particularly challenging for families (see Chapter 2). The child's temperament may affect his or her family's ability to cope with illness (Wallander, Hubert, & Varni, 1988). Furthermore, lower socioeconomic status appears to be associated with patterns of family interaction that can contribute to problems with psychological adjustment (Holmbeck et al., 2002).

Children and families coping with health conditions generally require support with psychosocial issues. It is important for clinicians to understand the impact that the illness has on the child and family with regard to the barriers presented, as well as their resources for coping with emerging challenges. This information can be useful in designing interventions to strengthen parent–child attachments and sibling relationships, and to resolve conflictual relationships that may arise.

Maintaining adaptive levels of family cohesion and strengthening family attachments throughout the course of an illness are important in promoting success in school. Parents who are strongly attached to their child and responsive to their child's needs are in a position to serve as effective advocates in the school. In addition, the quality of the parent–child relationship has been demonstrated to have an effect on the child's competence in school and peer relationships (Howes, Hamilton, & Matheson, 1994; Pianta & Harbers, 1996). Thus, building effective and supportive family relationships is a critical foundation for promoting successful school integration.

The capacity of the family to be responsive to the child and to promote effective school integration is affected by the relationship between the family and the healthcare system. It is important to understand this connection and to examine the extent to which the healthcare system strengthens family relationships or presents barriers to family coping and adjustment (Kazak & Simms, 1996). This information can be useful in designing interventions to promote more effective collaboration between the family and the healthcare system.

Preintegration: Step 2. Preparing the Family to Partner with the School

The second step in the process of integration is to prepare the family to engage in a partnership with the school. The importance of families and schools working together has been very well documented as a key factor in the educational success of children (e.g., Christenson & Sheridan, 2001; Pianta & Walsh, 1996). When addressing the needs of children with health problems, this partnership becomes even more critical. Given the enormous challenges these children face in school and the limited capacity that schools often have in addressing complex medical conditions, collaborating with the school can be a difficult and frustrating process for families. The challenges often are magnified in low-income communities in which the culture of the school is highly incongruent with the culture of the surrounding neighborhoods (Comer, Hayners, Joyner, & Ben-Avie, 1996). Parents typically are required to serve as strong advocates for their child, but this may result in family–school relationship patterns that are adversarial and mutually coercive (Power & Bartholomew, 1987).

Families need to understand school ecology, including the mission of schools, and public regulations that direct school policy. They need to learn about the culture of the schools in their community, as well as the resources and limitations of the schools to address complex health problems. Furthermore, it is important for families to know about resources in the community (e.g., healthcare and mental healthcare providers, community-based advocacy groups, and faith-based organizations) that can assist with school transitions.

Providing families with a framework for engaging in collaborative problem solving with educators also is critical to effective integration. In successful home–school relationships, parents and educators are colearners, coteachers, and co–decision makers (Christenson & Sheridan, 2001). Parents respect the authority of teachers in the school domain, and teachers respect the authority of parents in the home domain (Power & Bartholomew, 1987). Both parties are actively involved in educating themselves and supporting each other in learning useful strategies for nurturing the child's cognitive, social, and emotional development (see Christenson & Sheridan, 2001, for a description of specific strategies to promote successful family–school collaboration).

Preintegration: Step 3. Preparing Schools to Partner with the Family and Healthcare System

As families are being prepared to partner with schools, educational professionals need to be oriented about how to collaborate effectively with families to address the complex health needs of the child. Although some families have, or are able to develop, strategies for initiating a fruitful family–school partnership, it is typically the responsibility of school professionals to set the tone and create the context for a mutually supportive family–school collaboration (Christenson & Sheridan, 2001). To facilitate this process with children who have health problems, it is important for educators to understand the medical condition, the challenges to the child and family in coping with this condition, and the cognitive, social, and emotional needs of the child in the school context (Prevatt et al., 2000). Furthermore, teachers need to understand the significance of effective family–school collaboration and strategies for engaging families in effective partnerships to address the challenges these children face in school.

To assist children and families coping with medical problems, school professionals need to work effectively with health providers. Unfortunately, school personnel generally lack training and experience in collaborating with healthcare professionals (Power, Atkins, Osborne, & Blum, 1994). Differences between the school and healthcare system with regard to mission, culture, regulations governing practice, models of practice, and language can serve as obstacles to effective communication across systems. As a result of these barriers, school and healthcare professionals often fail to communicate, depriving children of the benefits of collaboration and leaving parents in the challenging position of being the spokesperson for each group. School professionals often need encouragement and guidance to initiate collaboration and to engage in effective partnerships with healthcare providers.

Integration: Step 4. Engaging the Family, School, and Health System in a Collaborative Process

Once all the systems involved with the child have been prepared, the actual consultative process can begin. This step offers the greatest challenge for professionals in promoting effective school integration. Collaboration across systems is required to design, implement, and evaluate specific strategies to promote the child's cognitive and social competence in school. Conjoint behavioral consultation (Sheridan, 1997; Sheridan, Kratochwill, & Bergan, 1996) is a highly useful model for guiding the collaborative, problem-solving process that can facilitate effective integration.

Conjoint Behavioral Consultation

Behavioral consultation (Bergan & Kratochwill, 1990) is a well-researched and well-developed process that focuses on solving student problems indirectly by providing consultation to individuals who are direct service providers (i.e., teachers and other school personnel). Behavioral consultation typically incorporates a functional behavioral assessment framework for conceptualizing and designing interventions to treat a wide range of school-based problems, including academic, behavioral, and social problems (Erchul & Martens, 1997; Galloway & Sheridan, 1994; Kratochwill, Elliott, & Busse, 1995). This consultation method involves a series of interviews with intervention participants to identify problems, collect and analyze functional assessment data, design an intervention plan, implement the intervention, and evaluate outcomes (Kratochwill & Bergan, 1990).

Although behavioral consultation generally is an effective approach for improving children's adaptation in schools, this set of procedures traditionally has focused primarily on providing consultation to school professionals alone. By so doing, the process may fail to capitalize on contributions that families can make in collaboration with educators to address children's educational needs (Christenson & Conoley, 1992; Christenson, Rounds, & Gorney, 1992; Pianta & Walsh, 1996). Including families in the process has the potential to improve the effectiveness of behavioral consultation.

Recognizing the limitations of scope and setting of the behavioral consultation model, Sheridan et al. (1996) further developed this model so that it includes families and school professionals in the collaborative consultation process. Integrating ecological systems theory with the principles of behavioral psychology into the conceptual framework, conjoint behavioral consultation (CBC) incorporates the input of multiple informants in the family and school systems to understand the meaning and function of child behavior in each system. Furthermore, this approach seeks to elucidate how behaviors and processes occurring in one system have an impact on functioning in the other system.

Extensive research on CBC has been conducted over the past decade. Sheridan, Eagle, Cowan, and Mickelson (2001) reported the outcomes of 4 years of investigation in which CBC had been used to address a wide variety of problems. The reported CBC cases reflected consultation with 57 students, 53 parents, and 56 teachers. All of the cases involved collaborative consultation between school professionals and families. Students enrolled in this study were referred by school personnel for academic and/or behavioral problems. Results of their analyses found overall effect sizes across cases to range from 0.83 to 1.36, suggesting strong effects to CBC. Furthermore, their findings indicated that CBC was highly acceptable to participating parents and teachers.

CBC was designed to facilitate partnerships among other systems, in addition to the family and school, including the healthcare system and other community systems (e.g., mental healthcare system, child welfare system, juvenile justice system, and faith-based organizations; Sheridan et al., 1996). With children who have health conditions, CBC necessarily involves the integration of the family, school, and healthcare system in the problem-solving process. A brief outline of the steps involved in CBC is provided here. Readers interested in a comprehensive description of the model and process are referred to the manual written by Sheridan et al. (1996).

Stages of Conjoint Behavioral Consultation

Like behavioral consultation, CBC is divided into 4 stages. In the *problem identification* stage, the consultant and consultee work together to identify the key problem(s) to be targeted. However, because multiple systems are involved in the problem identification process, the assessment is much broader than that in behavioral consultation. For example, CBC usually includes a family assessment. The family assessment uses both interview and direct observation methods to determine family perspectives about presenting problems and to understand relationship patterns. During the interview, the consultant explores the family history and learns about parent–child and sibling interactions. The problem identification process often includes an interview with the target child, as well as the completion of self-report measures. The assessment should also include a functional assessment of behavior conducted in school and/or home settings. The purpose of the functional assessment is to identify factors contributing to the emergence and maintenance of problems with cognitive, social, and emotional adaptation (Haynes & O'Brien, 1990). This information can be highly useful in designing interventions tailored to address the specific needs of children and the challenges of families and school professionals.

The CBC problem identification interview is designed to address six goals: (1) establish working relationships among families, school professionals, and health providers; (2) specify the targets for intervention; (3) identify antecedent, situational, and consequent conditions for the targeted problems as part of a functional assessment; (4) determine the severity of the problems; (5) identify the goals of intervention; and (6) establish procedures for collecting baseline information. The inclusion of family members, school personnel, and healthcare professionals in the CBC process requires that the consultant be skilled in working effectively with individuals from each of these systems and in facilitating communications across systems.

The *problem analysis* stage of CBC involves an examination of baseline ecological and functional assessment data to design strategies that promote adaptive functioning within systems and that address the hypothesized functions of behavior. Intervention design should involve individuals from each system in the integration process (Sheridan et al., 1996). It is important for each stakeholder group, including the child and caregivers, school personnel, and healthcare professionals, to contribute to an interpretation of the assessment data and to share perspectives about the social validity of potential intervention plans. Social validity refers to stakeholder views about the appropriateness and acceptability of the goals, strategies, and intended outcomes of intervention (Kazdin, 1980; Schwartz & Baer, 1991). Intervention plans should reflect the priorities and values of participants from each system in order to increase the likelihood of intervention adherence and effectiveness (Reimers, Wacker, & Koeppl, 1987; Witt & Elliott, 1985).

The next step of CBC is *treatment implementation*. During this phase, the consultant ensures that participants in the intervention process understand their roles and receive the orientation needed to perform their responsibilities competently. Intervention integrity, which refers to the extent to which intervention strategies are implemented as designed, is a critical component of this phase. Strategies to improve integrity might include (1) providing systematic training to participants, (2) preparing written scripts to guide the implementation process, (3) using self-monitoring strategies to assist participants in directing their own work, and (4) arranging for a consultant or peer to observe intervention sessions (e.g., through the use of video and audio procedures or direct observations), then offering feedback to participants (Ernhardt, Barnett, Lentz, Stollar, & Reifin, 1996; Gresham, 1989).

In the final stage, *treatment evaluation*, the consultant and participants review outcome data to determine the extent to which the integration process is effective in achieving specified goals. Evaluation is conceived as both a formative and summative process. Outcome data are collected formatively during the course of school integration, so that adjustments can be made along the way. Also, outcomes are examined summatively after a designated time period to determine whether goals have been attained, and whether a revision of the integration plan is needed. Furthermore, the social validity of the intervention needs to be evaluated by determining the extent to which functioning has been "normalized" and the degree to which participants perceive the intervention to be acceptable.

APPLYING CBC TO INTEGRATING STUDENTS WITH HEALTH PROBLEMS

The CBC model provides a framework for (1) aligning the family, school, and healthcare systems to facilitate the integration of children with health problems into school and (2) integrating systems of care into the problem-solving process. Although this framework and set of methods generally have been demonstrated to be effective, the process is primarily problem-focused and oriented toward deficit reduction. A limitation of this approach is that it may fail to acknowledge and build on the strengths of the child and assets in the family, school, and healthcare systems, which may be highly useful in designing strategies to prevent further health risk and promote resilience in the school context.

Thus, we recommend an adaptation of CBC that incorporates problem-focused *and* strength-based approaches to assessment of intervention. In the initial "problem/asset identification phase," the consultant collaborates with intervention stakeholders to identify both problems encountered by the child in multiple settings and assets of the child, family, school, and healthcare providers to promote adaptation across settings. During the intervention planning phase, child and system assets are used strategically to address problem areas. Furthermore, strategies are developed to build child assets and to strengthen the systems to enable the child to become more resilient. Next, prevention strategies are implemented simultaneously with intervention approaches, so that problems get resolved while the child and the systems that support him or her are becoming increasingly stronger and more resilient. The outcomes of both prevention and intervention efforts are evaluated formatively, so that strategies can be adjusted during the change process. The following case illustrates a strength-based application of the CBC model.

Case of Jackson

Jackson, 11 years of age, was hospitalized after sustaining a moderate to severe closed head injury during a bike accident. After a 48-hour stabilization period, he was transferred to the neurorehabilitation unit of a children's hospital. Upon review of records, a neuropsychologist noted that, prior to the accident, Jackson had above average cognitive ability and was performing at an above average level in reading and at an average level in all other academic subjects. School records revealed a history of minor difficulties paying attention, following directions, and completing homework, although he had never been diagnosed with ADHD. The parents reported that he was a sensitive child who was prone to worry. There was no evidence of depression or significant conduct problems prior to injury.

A brief neuropsychological evaluation performed 7 days after the accident revealed an estimated Wechsler Intelligence Scale for Children—III (WISC-III) Verbal IQ in the above-average range and a Performance IQ in the borderline range. Significant problems with visual–spatial memory, visual–motor integration, and fine motor functioning were apparent. Further evidence of right-hemisphere involvement was suggested by relative weaknesses on fine motor tasks involving the left versus right hand. Performance on a continuous performance task and reports from hospital staff suggested significant problems with attention span and impulse control. Also, on two occasions, Jackson displayed temper outbursts with hospital staff when he could not have his way. Reports from his parents revealed that Jackson had two close friends in the neighborhood, and that he had well-developed art skills. During the early period of recovery, he demonstrated little interest in drawing and resisted efforts to engage him in art activities.

Jackson lived in a two-parent family with an 8-year-old brother and 6-year-old sister. Both parents worked full-time, and the children were placed in day care after school until a parent arrived to pick them up in the late afternoon. Although both parents reported a close relationship with Jackson, the father worked long hours, leaving little time for him to spend with his son. The mother assumed primary responsibility for school and homework issues, and household chores. She admitted that Jackson was challenging to parent and often argumentative at home. Jackson and his brother often fought; the relationship with the sister was generally cooperative.

During a family interview in the first week of hospitalization, the parents were very upset and expressed guilt that their failure to supervise Jackson's neighborhood activities closely may have contributed to the accident. To address Step 1 of preintegration, the consulting psychologist provided supportive counseling and conducted a family assessment with Jackson present. Several subsequent meetings with the family were also conducted. During one of these meetings, the consultant and the neuropsychologist met with the family to discuss the nature of the head injury, its short-term effects, and the expected course of recovery, including the range of prognoses. The consultant assisted family members in understanding the information and formulating questions about their concerns. The psychologist emphasized the importance of strengthening parent–child relationships as a first step of intervention. The parents were assisted in engaging Jackson in a dialogue about projects they could work on together during the hospitalization. They were encouraged to modify their work schedules to become more available to the child during this period. The consultant carefully observed the parents as they worked together and intervened to promote better communication and more adaptive problem solving.

Toward the end of the hospitalization, the psychologist met with the parents and child to discuss potential challenges Jackson might encounter upon reentry to school, thereby addressing Step 2 of preintegration. The challenges included increased problems with writing assignments, such as seatwork, homework, and tests; difficulty paying attention and listening to instruction in class; and problems with anger control. Assets of the child and resources of the school that would enable Jackson to address school challenges were identified. Jackson and his parents expressed a lack of trust toward the current teacher but indicated that the teacher from the previous year had a strong relationship with Jackson. Also, one of Jackson's best friends was in his class for most of the day. The parents were informed about Jackson's educational rights as a child with a handicapping condition and a disability.

With parent permission, the consultant contacted the principal and described Jackson's condition and the challenges he would likely encounter upon return to school (Step 3 of preintegration). The consultant provided the principal with written information about Jackson and requested that his teachers be briefed about his condition and its likely impact on school functioning. In addition, the consultant spoke with the principal about the need to involve the district's Department of Special Services to assist in the process of disability determination. A meeting at the school was scheduled for the parents, key school personnel, including the teacher from the previous year, and the hospital consultant.

At the family–school meeting (Step 4, integration), the consultant's initial goal was to establish the basis for a strong partnership involving the family, school, and healthcare team. Next, the psychologist facilitated a discussion to identify both potential child concerns in school (e.g., problems with work completion, attention, and anger control) and potential assets (e.g., close friend in the same class, supportive relationships with school staff, adequate verbal ability), as part of the problem/asset identification process. The psychologist described the findings of functional assessments of behavior during listening and seatwork tasks performed in the hospital, which revealed that the primary function of Jackson's behavior during these activities was task avoidance.

As a transition into the intervention planning phase, the psychologist highlighted the critical need to establish strong attachments for the child across all systems of functioning. The parents described some of the strategies they had been using in the hospital to strengthen their relationship with Jackson, which included spending time playing board and card games with him. School professionals were encouraged to think of ways to relate effectively with Jackson upon his return to school. Providing opportunities for Jackson to meet with last year's teacher and to receive assistance from his close friend in class were discussed. The school team and parents were then encouraged to consider accommodation strategies for assisting Jackson to listen to classroom instruction and to work on assigned written work, taking into account that his behavior during these activities was primarily designed to avoid demands. Strategies that included allowing Jackson a choice of work activities, reducing the duration of high-demand activities, and providing positive reinforcement contingent on paying attention and attaining realistic goals for productivity were discussed (see DuPaul & Ervin, 1996, for a description of interventions that address the different functions of behavior). Also, during the meeting, the family and school team agreed that Jackson should receive occupational therapy, and a schedule for providing this service was negotiated. An important goal of occupational therapy was to assist him in regaining interest in art activities. Furthermore, strategies to assist with attention in class and anger control were discussed. During the meeting, the roles of each member of the school and healthcare teams, as well as those of the parents and child, were specified to assist with intervention implementation.

For purposes of outcome evaluation, formative and summative outcomes were to be assessed by portfolio methods involving the review of tests, quizzes, seatwork and homework; teacher reports of child behavior and social skills; child report of anxiety and self-esteem; and peer reports of social acceptability. A written, individualized education plan that included target problems, assets and resources, intervention goals, strategies of intervention, outcome measures, and periods for reviewing outcome data was prepared. The family and school team met on a bimonthly basis for the initial 6 months to review progress and modify the intervention plan. Both parents were strongly encouraged to attend these meetings. The consultant attended the 2-month follow-up meeting and stayed in contact with the family and school team via telephone after that.

CONCLUSIONS

Fully integrating children with health problems into the fabric of the school can be a challenging process for the family, school professionals, and healthcare team. We recommend a four-step integration process based on principles of ecological systems theory and functional behavioral assessment. The first three steps are designed to prepare the family, school team, and healthcare team for integration, and the fourth step focuses on coordinating these systems to plan, implement, and evaluate strategies of integration. CBC provides a highly useful framework for achieving the fourth step in the process. A hallmark of the CBC approach is to involve stakeholders from all salient systems in the child's life in the process of designing, implementing, and evaluating the intervention program. Interventions are designed to enable the child to function more competently within each system and to promote collaborative working relationships among family members and professionals from the school and healthcare systems. In implementing CBC, we recommend an approach that integrates a strength-based, asset-building approach with one focused on deficit reduction and problem solving. In this way, efforts to build resilience and to prevent further health risk can be incorporated with strategies to address emerging challenges and problems.

REFERENCES

Benner, A. E., & Marlow, L. S. (1991). The effect of a workshop on childhood cancer on students' knowledge, concerns, and desire to interact with a classmate with cancer. *Children's Health Care, 20,* 101–107.

Bergan, J. R., & Kratochwill, T. R. (1990). *Behavioral consultation and therapy.* New York: Plenum Press.

Black, K. C., & Hynd, G. W. (1995). Epilepsy in the school age child: Cognitive-behavioral characteristics and effects on academic performance. *School Psychology Quarterly, 10,* 345–458.

Bronfenbrenner, U. (1979). *The ecology of human development.* Cambridge, MA: Harvard University Press.

Brown, R. T. (1995). Introduction to the special series: Cognitive and academic issues related to chronic illness. *School Psychology Quarterly, 10,* 271–273.

Carlson, C. I., Tharinger, D. J., Bricklin, P. M., DeMers, S. T., & Paavola, J. C. (1996). Health care reform and psychological practice in schools. *Professional Psychology: Research and Practice, 27,* 14–23.

Chekryn, J., Deegan, M., & Reid, J. (1987). Impact on teachers when a child with cancer returns to school. *Children's Health Care, 12,* 234–245.

Christenson, S. L., & Conoley, J. C. (Eds.). (1992). *Home–school collaboration: Enhancing children's academic and social competence.* Silver Spring, MD: National Association of School Psychologists.

Christenson, S. L., Rounds, T., & Gorney, D. (1992). Family factors and student achievement: An avenue to increase students's success. *School Psychology Quarterly, 7,* 178–206.

Christenson, S. L., & Sheridan, S. M. (2001). *Schools and families: Creating essential connections for learning.* New York: Guilford Press.

Clark, E., Russman, S., & Orme, S. (1999). Traumatic brain injury: Effects on school functioning and intervention strategies. *School Psychology Review, 28,* 242–250.

Comer, J. P., Haynes, N. M., Joyner, E. T., & Ben-Avie, M. (1996). *Rallying the whole village: The Comer process for reforming education.* New York: Teachers College Press.

DuPaul, G. J., & Eckert, T. (1994). The effects of social skill curricula: Now you see them, now you don't. *School Psychology Quarterly, 9,* 113–132.

DuPaul, G. J., & Ervin, R. A. (1996). Functional assessment of behaviors related to attention-deficit/hyperactivity disorder. *Behavior Therapy, 27,* 601–622.

Erchul, W. P., & Martens, B. K. (1997). *School consultation: Conceptual and empirical bases of practice.* New York: Plenum Press.

Ernhardt, K. E., Barnett, D. W., Lentz, F. E., Stollar, S. A., & Reifin, L. H. (1996). Innovative methodology in ecological consultation: Use of scripts to promote treatment acceptability and integrity. *School Psychology Quarterly, 11,* 149–168.

Farmer, J. E., & Peterson, L. (1995). Pediatric traumatic brain injury: Promoting successful school reentry. *School Psychology Review, 24,* 230–243.

Galloway, J., & Sheridan, S. M. (1994). Implementing scientific practices through case studies: Examples using home–school interventions and consultation. *Journal of School Psychology, 32,* 385–413.

Glang, A., Todis, B., Cooley, E., Wells, J., & Voss, J. (1997). Building social networks for children and adolescents with traumatic brain injury: A school-based intervention. *Journal of Head Trauma Rehabilitation, 12,* 32–47.

Gresham, F. M. (1989). Assessment of treatment integrity in school consultation and prereferral intervention. *School Psychology Review, 18,* 37–50.

Haynes, S. N., & O'Brien, W. H. (1990). Functional analysis in behavior therapy. *Clinical Psychology Review, 10,* 649–668.

Holmbeck, G., Coakley, R., Hommeyer, J., Shapera, W., & Westhoven, V. (2002). Observed and perceived dyadic and systemic functioning in families of preadolescents with spina bifida. *Journal of Pediatric Psychology, 27,* 177–189.

Holtzman, W. H. (Ed.). (1992). *School of the future.* Washington, DC: American Psychological Association.

Howes, C., Hamilton, C., & Matheson, C. (1994). Children's relationships with peers: Differential associations with aspects of the teacher–child relationship. *Child Development, 65,* 253–264.

Individuals with Disabilities Education Act—Amendments of 1997. (1997). U.S. Congress, Public Law 101–476; amended by Public Law 105–17.

Katz, E. R., Varni, J. W., Rubenstein, C. L., Blew, A., & Hubert, N. (1992). Teacher, parent, and child evaluative ratings of a school reintegration intervention for children with newly diagnosed cancer. *Children's Health Care, 21,* 69–75.

Kazak, A. (2001). Comprehensive care for children with cancer and their families: A social ecological framework guiding research, practice and policy. *Children's Services: Social Policy, Research and Practice, 4,* 217–233.

Kazak, A. E., Rourke, M. T., & Crump, T. A. (in press). Families and other systems in pediatric psychology. In M. C. Roberts (Ed.), *Handbook of pediatric psychology* (3rd ed.). New York: Guilford Press.

Kazak, A. E., Segal-Andrews, A. M., & Johnson, K. (1995). Pediatric psychology research and practice: A family/systems approach. In M. C. Roberts (Ed.), *Handbook of pediatric psychology* (2nd ed., pp. 84–104). New York: Guilford Press.

Kazak, A. E., & Simms, S. (1996). Children with life-threatening illnesses: Psychological difficulties and interpersonal relationships. In F. Kaslow (Ed.), *Handbook of relational diagnosis and dysfunctional family patterns* (pp. 225–238). New York: Wiley.

Kazdin, A. E. (1980). Acceptability of alternative treatments for deviant child behavior. *Journal of Applied Behavior Analysis, 13,* 259–273.

Kratochwill, T. R., & Bergan, J. R. (1990). *Behavioral consultation in applied settings: An individual guide.* New York: Plenum Press.

Kratochwill, T. R., Elliott, S. N., & Busse, R. T. (1995). Behavioral consultation: A five-year evaluation of consultant and client outcomes. *School Psychology Quarterly, 10,* 87–117.

Kratochwill, T. R., & McGivern, J. E. (1996). Clinical diagnosis, behavioral assessment, and functional analysis: Examining the connection between assessment and intervention. *School Psychology Review, 25,* 342–355.

Mateer, C. A., Kerns, K. A., & Eso, K. L. (1997). Management of attention and memory disorders following traumatic brain injury. In E. D. Bigler, E. Clark, & J. E. Farmer (Eds.), *Childhood traumatic brain injury: Diagnosis, assessment, and intervention* (pp. 153–175). Austin, TX: Pro-Ed.

Phelps, L. (Ed.). (1998). *Health-related disorders in children and adolescents: A guidebook for understanding and educating.* Washington, DC: American Psychological Association.

Pianta, R. C. (2001). Implications of a developmental systems model for preventing and treating behavioral disturbances in children and adolescents. In J. N. Hughes, A. M. La Greca, & J. C. Conoley (Eds.), *Handbook for psychological services for children and adolescents* (pp. 23–42). New York: Oxford University Press.

Pianta, R. C., & Harbers, K. L. (1996). Observing mother and child behavior in a problem-solving situation at school entry: Relations with academic achievement. *Journal of School Psychology, 34,* 307–322.

Pianta, R. C., & Walsh, D. (1996). *High-risk children in the schools: Creating sustaining relationships.* New York: Routledge.

Power, T. J., Atkins, M. S., Osborne, M. L., & Blum, N. J. (1994). The school psychologist as manager of programming for ADHD. *School Psychology Review, 23,* 279–291.

Power, T. J., & Bartholomew, K. L. (1987). Family-school relationship patterns: An ecological assessment. *School Psychology Review, 14,* 222–229.

Prevatt, F. F., Heffer, R. W., & Lowe, P. A. (2000). A review of school reintegration programs for children with cancer. *Journal of School Psychology, 38,* 447–467.

Rehabilitation Act of 1973. (1973). U.S. Congress, Public Law 93–112.

Reimers, T. M., Wacker, D. P., & Koeppl, G. (1987). Acceptability of behavioral interventions: A review of the literature. *School Psychology Review, 16,* 212–227.

Riccio, C. A., & Hughes, J. N. (2001). Established and emerging models of psychological services in school settings. In J. N. Hughes, A. M. La Greca, & J. C. Conoley (Eds.), *Handbook of psychological services for children and adolescents* (pp. 63–88). New York: Oxford University Press.

Roberts, M. C., & Hurley, L. K. (1997). *Managing managed care.* New York: Plenum Press.

Ross, J. W. (1984). Resolving non-medical obstacles to successful school reentry for children with cancer. *Journal of School Health, 54,* 84–86.

Schwartz, I. S., & Baer, D. M. (1991). Social validity assessments: Is current practice state of the art? *Journal of Applied Behavior Analysis, 24,* 189–204.

Sexon, S. B., & Madan-Swain, A. (1993). School re-entry for the child with chronic illness. *Journal of Learning Disabilities, 26,* 115–125, 137.

Sheridan, S. M. (1997). Conceptual and empirical bases of conjoint behavioral consultation. *School Psychology Quarterly, 12,* 119–133.

Sheridan, S. M., Eagle, J. W., Cowan, R. J., & Mickelson, W. (2001). The effects of conjoint behavioral consultation: Results of a 4–year investigation. *Journal of School Psychology, 39,* 361–385.

Sheridan, S. M., Kratochwill, T. R., & Bergan, J. R. (1996). *Conjoint behavioral consultation: A procedural manual.* New York: Plenum Press.

Short, R. J., & Talley, R. C. (1997). Rethinking psychology in the schools: Implications of recent national policy. *American Psychologist, 52,* 234–240.

Treiber, F. A., Schramm, L., & Mabe, P. A. (1986). Children's knowledge and concerns toward a peer with cancer: A workshop intervention approach. *Child Psychiatry and Human Development, 16,* 249–260.

Vannatta, K., Gertstein, M., Short, A., & Noll, R. (1998). A controlled study of peer relationships of children surviving brain tumors. *Journal of Pediatric Psychology, 23,* 279–287.

Wallander, J. L., Hubert, N. C., & Varni, J. W. (1988). Child and maternal temperament characteristics, goodness of fit and adjustment in handicapped children. *Journal of Clinical Psychology, 17,* 366–344.

Wallander, J. L., & Thompson, R. J. (1995). Psychosocial adjustment of children with chronic physical conditions. In M. C. Roberts (Ed.), *Handbook of pediatric psychology* (2nd ed., pp. 124–141). New York: Guilford Press.

Weitzman, M. (1986). School absence rates as outcome measures in studies of children with chronic illness. *Journal of Chronic Illness, 39,* 799–808.

Witt, J. C., & Elliott, S. N. (1985). Acceptability of classroom intervention strategies. In T. R. Kratochwill (Ed.), *Advances in school psychology* (Vol. 4; pp. 251–288). Hillsdale, NJ: Erlbaum.

Worchel-Prevatt, F. F., Heffer, R. W., Prevatt, B. C., Miner, J., Young-Saleme, T., Horgan, D., & Lopez, M. A. (1998). A school reentry program for chronically ill children. *Journal of School Psychology, 36,* 261–279.

CHAPTER 5

Promoting Intervention Adherence

Linking Systems to Promote Collaborative Management

With the advances seen in modern medicine, the expected linear sequence of events is that an illness is diagnosed and subsequently treated. The outcome, often but not always a cure, results from the accuracy and success of the diagnosis and treatments. Unfortunately, healthcare is rarely this simple, particularly when serious and chronic illnesses of childhood are considered. In some cases, issues as basic as access to healthcare and insurance coverage for treatment may hinder effective healthcare provision (U.S. Department of Health and Human Services, 1999). The diagnosis of illness and treatment is often intricate, and sometimes inaccurate or unsuccessful. Not all childhood illnesses can be cured: Some are fatal and many are chronic, with associated long-term functional impairment. In many cases, prevention is a reasonable and preferred goal.

Many factors may impact the successful treatment of children. These factors, and interventions to address them from a systems perspective, are the focus of this chapter. Rather than using a linear model (diagnosis → treatment → outcome), we advocate a more complex, systems-oriented approach. We assume the accuracy of diagnosis and concern ourselves with factors that contribute to successful treatment, in particular, intervention adherence. We reframe questions about adherence within a broader systemic model of collaborative management, requiring orchestration of efforts to enhance care across, in this case, the family, school, and healthcare teams.

Many of the diseases discussed in this chapter are chronic in nature and among the serious pediatric illnesses most commonly encountered by school personnel (e.g., asthma, obesity, diabetes, cancer). However, issues related to adherence are also relevant in acute illnesses and in common behavioral concerns, such as attention-deficit/hyperactivity disorder (ADHD). Finally, adherence to general health recommendations pertains to all children and has strong preventive implications. We provide general background on adherence and outline broad approaches for successful collaborations among patients, families, hospitals, and schools.

Pediatric illnesses themselves and their treatments pose many demands that often define the daily lives of children and families, and can determine the health outcomes. These may often include regimens for medications, exercise, and diet. The implications for adhering to treatment are often daunting (e.g., the child's life may be threatened, or other serious health concerns may be associated with nonadherence). These demands, and the implications of successful adherence, demand a coordinated response across settings in the child's life. While recognizing the always stressful and sometimes extraordinary demands of treatment on children families, schools, and healthcare systems, it is important to highlight their competence; that is, most patients and families adapt and cope with the demands of childhood illness, and most develop successful collaborative relationships to ensure their child's treatment and enhance health outcomes. Similarly, school and healthcare teams generally are competent, and bring considerable and varied resources to bear in successful treatment.

ADHERENCE: DEFINITIONS AND PREDICTORS

Illnesses vary widely along a number of factors, including onset, course, complications, severity, likely outcome, and treatment recommendations. Fortunately, some form of treatment is recommended for virtually all pediatric illnesses, many with very high likelihood of curing or controlling diseases that might otherwise pose severe and chronic threat to the lives and well-being of affected children. Although the stakes are often high, with successful outcome contingent on effective delivery of treatment, many complicated issues affect the successful treatment of childhood illness. How treatment recommendations are received and implemented by patients and families, and factors that affect the extent to which success is achieved, is the topic of the current chapter.

The Limitations of Existing Language: Compliance and Adherence

By asking whether treatment recommendations were received and implemented, we reframe and rephrase a common question—"Did the patient follow the prescribed treatment?" Although this appears to be a simple, albeit important question, responses suggest that it can be a highly complex issue. In our work, we reframe the question to shift the balance from one of patient compliance with medical orders to one that redistributes the responsibility across the ecology of the child patient and his or her social world. This is an essential reframing. Our premise in this chapter extends the concept, highlighting active partnerships among all stakeholders involved to achieve adherence.

Compliance was defined by Haynes (1979, pp. 2–3) as "the extent to which a person's behavior . . . coincides with medical or health advice." The use of the term "compliance" suggested a unilateral relationship (e.g., healthcare provider determines what patient should do) and assumed that the prescribed medical advice represents a "gold standard" that is understandable and important to the patient and family, reasonable to implement, and effective for all patients. The danger exists that the patient's and/or parent's perspective is not considered, and that only two options are obvious: to follow the advice or to be noncompliant. Although the term "compliance" continues to be used regularly in medical settings, an alternative—adherence—is preferred by many healthcare researcher and providers. As Riekert and Drotar (2000) note, adherence deemphasizes patient and family obedience and highlights the critical, active roles that patients and families play in treatment decisions. These issues are particularly salient in pediatrics in which the child is generally inseparable from the family.

Others have suggested more patient-oriented terms such as "self-care" and "disease management" (La Greca, 1990), and "self-regulation," "self-change," and "collaborative management" (Creer, 2000). In this chapter, we use these terms interchangeably. However, we endorse a model that is child- and family-centered, and one in which patient, family, healthcare team, school, and community are actively engaged with one another in pursuit of the goal of adaptive health outcomes. We refer to this as "collaborative management."

Prevalence and Implications of Nonadherence

Nonadherence is very common. In child healthcare, it is perhaps the rule and not the exception. A simple reflection on general adherence to health recommendations quickly provides a picture of the potential magnitude of these concerns; that is, to what extent are people in the general population completely adherent with recommendations regarding dental care? How often are all prescribed antibiotics used? Do people consistently follow dietary and exercise recommendations when weight may be complicating general health? Estimates of nonadherence specific to pediatric chronic illness vary widely, although reports in the range of 40–60% are common (Riekert & Drotar, 2000). A discussion of measurement issues in adherence is beyond the scope of this chapter, but it is not difficult to imagine the challenges in measuring whether a particular patient is adherent to treatment recommendations (Drotar, 2000).

Adherence is often conceptualized as whether or not a child has taken a medication. This simple dichotomous outcome is subject to error. The medication may need to be taken several times a day. Skipping a dose may be more or less significant, depending on the illness and its stage, and the patient may not understand this. There may be more than one medication, possibly on an alternate dosing schedule. There may be conflicting or unclear directives for what the patient and family should do if a dose is missed.

In many cases, adherence may pertain to several treatment recommendations, such as physical therapy, medication, diet, and/or restrictions in activity. For each, a clear dichotomous outcome may be unrealistic. How much physical therapy, for example, is necessary? What if one aspect of a diet is followed and another is disregarded?

Although thoughtful and sophisticated measurement approaches to adherence continue to be developed, the actual prevalence rates of nonadherence may be less relevant than their implications (Lemanek, Kamps, & Chung, 2001). The consequences of nonadherence include increased morbidity (disease symptoms and complications) and mortality. In addition, higher rates of healthcare utilization (e.g., more hospital visits) may lead to higher insurance premiums. And nonadherence may affect outcomes in clinical trials, rendering inaccurate data on the types and doses of interventions actually delivered.

Understanding and Predicting Adherence

In order to promote collaborative management of pediatric illnesses, we must understand factors associated with the likelihood of treatment adherence and, simultaneously, obstacles to successful collaborative management. A large literature exists from which some common findings can be extracted.

Bauman (2000) distinguishes two types of adherence—volitional and inadvertent. In volitional nonadherence, patients understand what is expected in terms of their medical regimen, but they knowingly do not follow the recommendations. In cases of inadvertent nonadherence, patients believe that they are following treatment recommendations but in fact may have inaccurate information or beliefs that pose additional obstacles (e.g., believing that one can follow treatment recommendations *and* skip doses or change regimens without penalty to their health). These categories are further complicated for children and adolescents; that is, depending on the child's age and developmental level, the responsibility for collaborative management is shared among family members. Misunderstandings or volitional nonadherence at the parental level will impact the child's behavior. Similarly, children and, in particular, adolescents may be nonadherent despite parental efforts to instill compliance behaviors.

Bauman (2000) outlines several risk factors for these two types of nonadherence. For example, the length, intensity, extent, and disruptiveness of the medical regimen may influence adherence. Some children and parents may feel that the demands of testing for blood sugars and injecting insulin several times a day may be too difficult and intrusive. Children and teens may resist regimens that make them feel different from peers. Closely related to the demand of the protocol are side effects of medication. It is natural to want to avoid the negative side effects of treatment and to engage in behaviors designed to escape them (e.g., flushing chemotherapy down the toilet). This can result in serious treatment implications.

It is also not uncommon to find that children and adolescents and their families may question the efficacy of the treatments. It may be difficult, for example, for a child to see that chemotherapy that makes him or her ill in the short run will be helpful in the long-term treatment of cancer. Parents may feel that some treatments are more important than others and advocate less stringently for some. This links to the underlying core beliefs of family members. If one believes that a health problem is uncontrollable, one may be less likely to comply with treatment, believing the adverse outcome is inevitable.

Some parents believe that their children should use as little medication as possible and may resist its use. As an example of conflicting beliefs between families and healthcare providers, cultural, spiritual, and/or religious beliefs may be in direct conflict with medical recommendations (e.g., blood transfusions in the case of Jehovah's Witnesses, belief in alternative treatment approaches).

When beliefs among families, the healthcare team, and school personnel clash, a key factor in adherence emerges—lack of collaboration among the three parties. A large literature on physician–patient communication highlights many ways in which relationships affect outcome in medical care. Differences in expectations in terms of the types of information to be exchanged are common, as are imbalances in the perspective, power, and style of patients and healthcare providers (Korsch & Harding, 1997). Particularly with the increase in highly technological medical care, the need for trust and effective communication among patients, families, and healthcare providers is essential. Parents are encouraged to take an active role in the care of their child and often coordinate care and facilitate communication among all parties. Some parents are able to assume this role and function very effectively in it. Others are unable, or uncomfortable, doing so. In pediatric healthcare, the family-centered care movement has outlined a strong philosophy and many related resulting recommendations that reinforce the important role of families in assisting with the healthcare of their children (Johnson, 2000).

Nonadherence, or the failure of collaborative management, is upsetting to all parties. Patterns of parent–child interaction can easily become negative, because conflicts within families may further complicate following medical regimens. For staff members in hospitals and schools alike, it is disturbing when treatment recommendations are not followed. Particularly in the case of potentially life-threatening situations, conflicts among families, healthcare providers, and schools frequently escalate when treatment may appear to be undermined. At worst, conflicts erupt throughout the system and can escalate (e.g., when referrals are made to external agencies, such as social welfare or legal entities, in order to enforce the provision of treatment).

Limitations in Existing Approaches to Adherence

It is helpful in considering the broader context of treatment adherence to reflect on some of the limitations of existing models. From the perspective of the healthcare team, successful treatment of the child's illness is the major concern. Although family-centered care encourages compassionate consideration of the family's broader context, the role that illness plays in the family's life is sometimes overlooked; that is, managing illness is only one of the many challenges faced by the child and family. A systems-oriented view of adherence encourages an understanding that different members of the team (patient, family, healthcare providers, schools) may have divergent views of the relative importance of adherence behaviors.

Another limitation of existing views of adherence is the relatively scant recognition given to the fact that patients and families may work very hard to control a chronic illness (e.g., follow intensive and extensive treatment recommendations), yet find that their lives are not necessarily better. By its very nature, chronic illness is generally not curable. Individuals and families may maintain their quality of life but feel discouraged when their efforts do not necessarily improve their lives beyond the constraints of their health conditions.

Most of the literature on adherence is correlational, identifying variables associated with measures of adherence, which may include biological markers, self-report scales, parent report, or medical staff report data. Relatively little research has been conducted in terms of interventions to enhance adherence, particularly in terms of translating studies to important settings in the child's life, including the home, community, and school.

Finally, many discussions of adherence convey a sense that a child's and family's adherence status is stable; the reality is that adherence is likely to fluctuate markedly. Shortly after a diagnosis of asthma in a child, the family may be motivated to adhere to medication and environmental recommendations. As the child's illness appears to be in good control, this diligence may wax and wane. Relatedly, as the child grows older, adherence may become worse when the older child is in more environments in which parental control over allergens cannot be monitored.

A SYSTEMS MODEL OF COLLABORATIVE MANAGEMENT
Social Ecology

In order to illustrate a systems-oriented model for collaborative management in pediatric health, we draw on the social-ecological model that has been applied to pediatric illness (Kazak, Segal-Andrews, & Johnson, 1995). Based upon the work of Bronfrenbrenner (1979), the social-ecological model (Figure 5.1) provides a context for understanding interactions among childhood illnesses and the individuals and systems affected. It offers a framework to organize how children, families, healthcare settings, and schools interact with regard to commonplace issues, such as adherence. In this chapter we emphasize the child, family, healthcare settings, and school.

The Child

In social ecology, the child is at the center of a series of concentric circles. The child's circle is nested within a larger circle that includes members of the family system (mothers, fathers, siblings, extended family) and the illness (type, course, prognosis, chronicity). The child, illness, and family members interact with one another continuously. For example, children must have parental consent to initiate treatment and, even for adolescents, family members assume substantial responsibility for ensuring

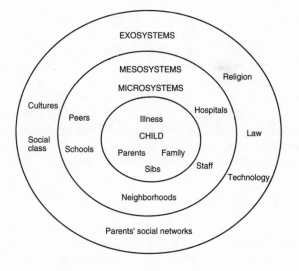

FIGURE 5.1. The social ecology of pediatric chronic illness. Adapted from Kazak, Segal-Andrews, and Johnson (1995). Copyright 1995 by The Guilford Press. Adapted by permission.

compliance to treatment recommendations. The family has a broad and powerful impact throughout the course of treatment. Most of what is known about child adjustment to illness focuses on the individual child and his or her family.

As in developmental psychology more broadly, social ecology is concerned with growth and development. A key concept is that reciprocal interactions provide the context for growth. Just as infants and young children learn and grow from their interactions with their caregivers, so too do children with illnesses continue to grow and develop as they adjust to and cope with their health-related concerns. In the diagnosis of a childhood illness, there is always risk for developmental arrests; that is, as families cope and adjust to the realities of their child's health concerns, they may treat the child differently. This is not unexpected on a short-term basis. A child who is not feeling well physically may behave like a younger child, may be excused from some normal, developmentally appropriate expectations, and may seek comfort in the same manner as a younger child. However, the child should be expected to participate in treatment in a developmentally appropriate manner. The child and family reorganize around the illness, perhaps in a new configuration (e.g., people in the family may shift in their roles), and with a common goal of achieving successful treatment.

In this way, the characteristics of the child (including age) become important determinants of how a collaborative treatment plan will be implemented. Is the child, for example, of an age such that he or she can monitor the types and amounts of food eaten? What types of developmentally appropriate strategies might be used to help the child learn about the treatment regimen and the reasons for adhering to treatment? Can the child complete subcutaneous injections with supervision, or alone? Can the adolescent attend some medical appointments without family members, make treatment decisions, provide informed consent for participating in research studies, and so on?

The Illness and Treatment

The illness and its treatment are located within the innermost circle of the social ecology framework, because characteristics of illness and treatment affect the overall course of collaborative management. Diseases and treatment differ vastly and can assume different roles within the family context. Rolland (1994) describes a psychosocial typology of illness that includes consideration of onset (gradual, sudden), course (constant, accelerating, relapsing), outcome (death, survival), and degree of incapacitation. Considering each of these parameters provides an understanding of how illnesses may be affecting the patient and family members. Within each general type of medical condition (e.g., cancer, diabetes, epilepsy), there may be variability with regard to these psychosocial parameters. Illnesses also have their own developmental trajectories. Particularly in childhood, with the changes characteristic of development, the nature of the illness and its impact may shift over time as well.

Illnesses also vary in terms of their severity, although it is more difficult than might be expected to characterize severity. Some conditions are highly visible (e.g., cerebral palsy, amputation), whereas others cannot be discerned visually, unless the child is acutely ill (diabetes, epilepsy). Although sometimes considered counterintuitive, illness severity generally is not associated with adjustment, although it may affect the demands placed on the child and family for treatment. An exception is the case in which the child's illness impacts the central nervous system (CNS); that is, the added complexity of caring for children with neurocognitive impairments is associated consistently with more family difficulties (Wade, Taylor, Drotar, Stancin, & Yeates, 1996). More subjective factors (e.g., what the patient and family believe about the illness and its treatment) are generally more powerful predictors of outcome than relatively objective measures (e.g., physician ratings of the toxicity of the treatment; Kazak, Stuber, et al., 1998).

Families

A large body of research on families and childhood illness exists and may be summarized by examining some of the consistent predictors of well-being. These include, for example, family flexibility, integration into a supportive social network, being able to balance the demands of the illness with other family needs and responsibilities, clear family boundaries, effective communication, positive attributions, active coping, and the encouragement of development of individuals within the family (Kazak, 2001).

The research of Kazak and colleagues, among others, has contributed to an emphasis on the competencies of families as they cope with childhood handicaps and illnesses. Across a series of studies (see Kazak, 2001, for a summary), these researchers found that families with an affected child were more alike than different from nonaffected families, with only a subset demonstrating psychosocial difficulties at a clinical level. This is not meant to imply that families do not require or benefit from additional assistance, but rather underscores the competence of parents and families to become partners in the development and delivery of interventions in child health. These researchers have shown, for example, positive outcomes of interventions for procedural pain that incorporate parents in helping to reduce the distress of their child with leukemia (Kazak, Penati, Brophy, & Himelstein, 1998). Furthermore, they demonstrated the feasibility and helpfulness of an intervention that combines cognitive-behavioral and family therapy approaches for reducing symptoms of posttraumatic stress in survivors of childhood cancer (Kazak et al., 1999). Parent involvement, including incorporating parents in the written dissemination of an intervention (e.g., Kazak & Sorkin, 1997), underscores the important role of parents and families in enhancing treatment outcomes.

With respect to adherence, the role that families play may be indirect. Using the example of childhood asthma, Fiese and Wamboldt (2000) described family rituals as a potentially mediating factor in treatment adherence. Family rituals describe a broad range of family behavior, from highly structured religious activities to daily household routines (e.g., family meals; bedtime routines; sports activities; participation in events with extended family, neighbors, or community members). Family rituals may help families in maintaining disease-related treatment regimens indirectly by helping to reduce anxiety in family members, increase predictability, or help families adapt and apply effective problem solving to new demands. Fiese and Wamboldt (2000) note that there are many different types of families and family rituals, and they encourage the development of research to identify types of rituals that promote adherence for subgroups of families.

Another family characteristic that may impact adherence is parenting style. Davis and colleagues (2001) found that parental warmth, support, and control were associated with adherence in preschool- and school-age children with diabetes. These data are quite intriguing given the associations among parent–child conflict and adherence difficulties in adolescents with diabetes (e.g., Jacobson et al., 1994). The findings suggest the importance of understanding the role of parenting, and its changes over time, in disease management.

Most interventions for children with chronic illness have focused either on the child in isolation (e.g., cognitive-behavioral interventions), or they have included members of the family system (e.g., parent education). Using the example of adherence, most interventions to increase use of pediatric inhalers in asthma, for example, have focused on education for children and families. Consistent with our systems-oriented model, many other components of the social ecology are of critical importance.

Schools

For children, schools are essential elements of the ecology and are systems that interact with other systems (e.g., families, hospitals, communities), and it is these interactions that are central to the social-ecological model. Returning to the example of asthma, school-based programs for asthma education have been developed and evaluated (cf. Horner, 1998; Persaud et al., 1996). However, integration of the approaches to adherence across the child, family, and school is rare. Most hospital-based healthcare providers do not explicitly consider how treatment recommendations will be communicated to the child's school. These communications often happen between families and schools, perhaps including the child, but generally without considering approaches that would build on the strengths of all three systems in pursuing the common goal of the child's health.

Most literature on family–school relationships has not focused specifically on health-related issues. For example, Power and Bartholomew (1987) described five types of interaction styles between schools and families (avoidant, competitive, merged, one-way, and collaborative). These patterns can be applied to relationships between schools and hospitals, and hospitals and families. The need to integrate three systems amplifies the complications and underscores the challenges of three-way collaboration. For example, a family–school relationship may be avoidant, and the hospital–school relationship might be one-way. In this case, the school might look to the hospital for guidance on an asthma treatment plan, but the school and family do not have a solid, collaborative relationship. The family may fail to attend meetings or indicate that there are no problems with the current plan. Or, in the case of a competitive school–family relationship, the school may feel that they have better ways of controlling the asthma than the family (e.g., suspect that there is smoking in the home). These situations are ripe for misunderstanding, conflict, and adverse outcomes.

Peers

Another essential system that interacts with the child, family, and healthcare system, and directly overlaps with the school, is the peer system. Peers are critical in the process of socialization and recognized within the pediatric psychology literature as influential in terms of affecting the behavior of children, and of adolescents in particular. Peers are generally invisible in healthcare settings, whereas they are central in educational environments, thus providing an optimal area in which to link the healthcare and school ecologies. Traditionally, studies of peers in pediatric illness have focused on the role of peers in understanding the socialization of children with chronic illness such as cancer (Noll, LeRoy, Bukowski, Rogosch, & Kulkarni, 1991) and sickle-cell disease (Noll, Vannatta, Koontz, & Kalinyak, 1996), a literature that has generally underscored the normalcy of children with chronic illness while also highlighting some increased risk for social isolation. Using analogue studies, factors that influence peer acceptance and understanding have highlighted the strength of same-gender alliances and show that elementary school children do not necessarily change behavior based on information about medical reasons for obesity (Bell & Morgan, 2000) or consider severity of symptoms highly in their appraisal of peers (Guite, Walker, Smith, & Garber, 2000). More recent emphasis on the role of peers and health-risk behaviors provides promising new opportunities for interventions in schools. For example, La Greca and colleagues showed that risk-taking behaviors varied by peer crowd affiliation (e.g., whether one was in one of six self-nominated groups—popular, jocks, brains, burnouts, nonconformist, other) and that most high school students' friends belong to the same peer crowd (La Greca, Prinstein, & Fetter, 2001).

The Healthcare System

Given the prominence of the healthcare system in understanding adherence, it is surprising how little has been written describing models of hospital–family collaboration. Family-centered care is perhaps the most widely described (e.g., Johnson, 2000), with its clearly articulated principles affirming the importance and role of families in pediatric healthcare. This model is also widely accepted, with many of its recommendations (e.g., expanded roles for families with hospitals, parents employed by healthcare facilities, on-site family resource centers) implemented in children's hospitals nationwide.

Another movement advocating for the collaboration of families and healthcare teams in patient care is the Collaborative Family Healthcare Association (CFHA; *www.cfha.org*). With its mission highlighting collaboration, "the collaborative family healthcare model envisions seamless collaboration between psychosocial, biomedical, nursing and other healthcare providers. It views patient, family, community and provider systems as equally important participants in the healthcare process" (*www.cfha.org/model.asp*). In addition, the CFHA emphasizes the potential for this collaborative care model to impact on fiscal resources; that is, a coordinated, collaborative approach, viewing clinical medicine from a biopsychosocial framework, may be translated into economic outcomes by reducing duplicative care, by treating medical issues in isolation from psychosocial ones, and by building on the adaptive competencies of patients and families.

Most literature on parent–physician interaction has focused on the conflicts in the relationship and typically proposes approaches that can mitigate against the escalation of these tensions. There are data that show, for example, that pediatricians view verbal, cooperative, and compliant mothers more positively than those who demonstrate fewer of these attributes (Tellerman & Medio, 1993). This may be viewed as a training issue, in that pediatricians often do not have the skills or training necessary to deal with families they find difficult, and may not utilize some of the relatively simple steps that can facilitate these relationships (Sunde, Mabe, & Josephson, 1993). Cohen and Wamboldt (2000) present intriguing data, based on audiotaped speech samples of descriptions of parents of children with asthma and their asthma specialists, each talking about their perceptions of family–physician relationships. They found relationship difficulties in 15–40% of these interactions.

Waters (2001) described the lack of attention to relationship aspects of the doctor–patient–family interaction (relative to the focus on the purely medical aspects) as "medicine's dirty secret." Noting that the lack of attention to the relationship aspects of medicine are widely known but not discussed, Waters noted that collaborative models of healthcare are revolutionary in offering a solution to this imbalance. In advocating the practice of a family systems model in pediatric healthcare, tasks that are common to families and to staff can be identified, including soothing oneself in the face of stress, developing trust (in the relationships one must form to ensure optimal healthcare), and managing the inevitable conflicts that arise in modern healthcare (Kazak, Simms, & Rourke, 2002). Using this framework, a clinical protocol is proposed that guides a consultant to help the healthcare team address situations in which relationships between families and providers may become strained.

Family/Patient—Healthcare Team—School Triad

Collaborative management is the outcome of coordinated responses across the social ecology to treatment demands; that is, in order for treatment recommendations to be implemented successfully, they must be integrated across the family, healthcare, and school systems. If a child's disease is managed well at home and in the hospital but not at school, the outcome will not be successful. Similarly, if the school and family attempt to implement treatment recommendations in isolation from the medical team, they are doing so without the crucial expertise of the healthcare team. On some occasions, the healthcare team and school collaborate, but the family is isolated from these conversations, perhaps because they are seen as uninvolved or uncooperative. This is obviously problematic.

The coordination of care across systems is required for effective treatment. This is easier said than done and has implications for a model of adherence that differs from most predominant approaches. In the following section, we highlight specific pediatric health problems frequently encountered in schools. For each, we highlight general intervention strategies and illustrate how collaborative management can be implemented using a systems model.

In applying the social-ecological framework to childhood illness and collaborative management, we focus on the triad of the family/ patient (child, adolescent), the healthcare team, and the school team (see Figure 5.2). All three share a common commitment to promoting the well-being of the child, and all by necessity play critical roles in how illnesses are treated, and health and well-being promoted. Many factors may influence the way in which the triad functions. The three are rarely *explicitly* considered interactive partners in this endeavor and equal investors in a positive outcome (adherence).

Using the example of a school-age child with cancer, prior to the child's diagnosis, the child, school, and family are likely to have a relationship organized around the child's performance in school. The relationship may fluctuate around demands placed on the child, the child's success in school, occasional behavioral concerns, parental follow-through with requests made by the school, and family satisfaction with teachers. During the child's medical evaluation, the family becomes rap-

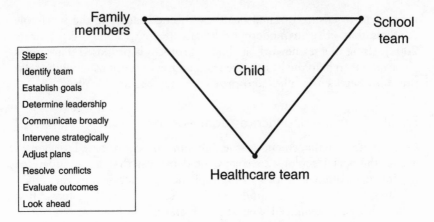

FIGURE 5.2. Steps to establishing and maintaining collaborative relationships among the family, healthcare team, and school team.

idly immersed in the healthcare system, usually necessitating the involvement of specialists, possible travel to new healthcare settings, and decision making about crucial treatment decisions. This represents an important change in the existing system, the loss of a previously healthy child, and the beginning of a new set of relationships organized around the child's illness and treatment. Until the point of diagnosis and determination of the treatment plan, the family is typically the conduit for information (e.g., explaining why the child is out of school). Once the child is medically stable and treatment is under way, the child/family–school–healthcare team triad must refocus to engage in collaborative management.

Understanding that the course of events that unfold during a child's treatment is unique and influenced by many variables, it is nonetheless instructive to illustrate some typical ways in which collaborative management unfolds, both adaptively and in situations in which conflict escalates. Adherence to childhood cancer treatment is often translated to mean "taking chemotherapy," specifically, taking pills, shots, and other treatments. In reality, it is much broader. Indeed, parents are often encouraged to help their child lead as normal a life as possible. A normal life includes going to school, functioning within one's peer group, and remaining actively engaged in a developmentally expected manner. Although children, families, schools, and healthcare providers typically agree with this plan, a systems-oriented approach to collaborative management might entail several specific steps that are often overlooked. Our premise is that consideration of these issues can provide a framework for anticipating and resolving problems. Most importantly, they may help ensure a positive adaptation to the illness and increased sense of self-efficacy across the major domains of the child's life.

A Systems-Oriented Protocol for Collaborative Management

The range of pediatric health conditions seen in communities and schools in the United States is vast. Increasingly, children with complicated health concerns are expected to function competently within community and school settings (Power, Heathfield, McGoey, & Blum, 1999). The added complexity of successfully implementing sophisticated treatments across settings and over time poses many challenges.

In this section, we outline briefly ways in which collaborative management can be approached. These guidelines are intended to be applicable across diseases and types of family, school, and healthcare systems. Both healthcare teams and school personnel generally look to parents for information regarding the child's health. Parents often are expected to assume a high level of responsibility for reporting to the school and health teams about the child's progress. This system may work reasonably well when the child's course of treatment proceeds smoothly. However, with children who have complex medical needs, the challenges of coping in the community can be monumental, and the responsibility for coordinating communications can be overwhelming. Using a collaborative management model, we suggest that the family, school, and healthcare team interact on multiple levels to coordinate care. There are several steps to this process and no right or wrong solutions to the questions posed. The steps vary with specific circumstances but represent important considerations in facilitating collaborative management.

Identify Team

The family, school, and healthcare teams have been discussed in the broadest possible manner. Yet at the point at which these parties come together to work on behalf of the child's health and well-being, identification of key membership of the collaborative team is necessary. Surprisingly, many stymied efforts at collaborative management can be traced to a lack of clarity in terms of the key team members. Who is in the family? What family members will be responsible for working with the school and hospital in ensuring the child's care across settings? Similarly, who from the healthcare team will be the primary contact person? Which school personnel will be involved, and how will their involvement (e.g., classroom teacher, guidance counselor, nurse) be clarified and coordinated? What will be child's role be?

Determine Leadership

Complex teams require that the roles of members be clearly defined while allowing for flexibility. When diverse stakeholders come together, there are often unspoken rules about who will lead the group. On some occasions, no one is clearly identified or supported to provide leadership. Many failures in collaborative management may be traced to a lack of clarity in terms of who is in charge of specific aspects of the collaboration. Who will gather information to assess whether the child's treatments are successful? Are there difficulties in home or school that affect the child's health? Who decides when a plan needs revision?

Establish Goals

It is helpful for the team to agree on the goals of collaboration at the outset. The conjoint behavioral consultation model outlined in Chapter 4 may be useful with problem identification and goal setting. What brings the team together to work on the child's behalf? For a child with a newly diagnosed condition, it may be applying well-established procedures (e.g., dispensing stimulant medications to a child with ADHD). For a child with asthma, it may be disseminating information about the child's use of an inhaler or increasing awareness of environmental triggers, and establishing what responsibility the child, teacher, and family have for the use of the intervention. Anticipation of future challenges should be included.

Communicate Broadly

At the outset, it is helpful to establish what information should be shared, with whom, and how. Parents may be unsure of what (and how much) to tell school personnel. School staff may feel uncertain as to how to get answers to their questions. School personnel see different sides of the child and can contribute valuable information that may not be as apparent to the family or healthcare team. Healthcare providers typically assume that, unless parents tell them, there are no school-related issues needing attention. Clearly specified channels of communication can facilitate the sharing of information and help those involved in the child's well-being obtain more information as needed. It can also help avert the development of a more antagonistic and conflictual relationship in which blame may be assigned (e.g., "The hospital was no help," "The family was not willing to give us what we needed," "The teacher didn't understand the importance of this").

Intervene Strategically

The heart of collaborative management is providing the appropriate intervention to facilitate the child's healthcare and well-being. Ideally, the different components of the systems involved should be working in an orchestrated, connected manner and avoid becoming isolated and disengaged from other parts of the systems. How can each party (school, healthcare team, parents, child) help meet the goals associated with the child's treatment? As is often the case, the child may have increased anxiety about visits to the hospital clinic, or may have problems with pain. How might the school help with these issues? What suggestions can be provided by parents and/or the healthcare team that could facilitate the child's well-being? Would it be helpful to use any of the established strategies for adherence?

Adjust Plans

Given the fluidity of systems and the constant developmental progress inherent in working with children, the need for change and adjustment in collaborative management plans is inevitable. When things go astray, what can be done? Some problems related to adherence are chronic. As will be shown later in this chapter, effective interventions can be implemented for many of these problems. Their effectiveness, however, depends on a plan that includes all relevant members of the social ecology and a coordinated effort to implement interventions. Without this collaboration, changes are unlikely to be satisfying and sustained.

Resolve Conflicts

There are always differences in perspectives and desired outcomes. Collaboration among three systems (family, school, hospital) makes some degree of conflict inevitable. A system of collaborative management includes a means by which disagreements among the team members can be resolved to avoid blame and defensiveness.

Look Ahead

It is tempting to remain focused on an immediate problem and its solution. Much of the frustration involved in improving adherence stems from the difficulty of sustaining changes. Although a treatment may be proceeding smoothly, given that children, illnesses, treatments, and systems change, what is likely to happen in a month, a year, or 5 years for this child's healthcare and with regard to subsequent education? What mechanisms can be developed in order to ensure that changes will be sustained? What role can families and schools play in helping children with serious and/or chronic illness grow into young adulthood with mastery of their healthcare needs?

Evaluate Outcomes

Knowing whether the established goals were met is essential in evaluating collaborative management (see Chapter 6 for a further discussion of outcome evaluation). Collecting data about outcomes is strongly recommended (e.g., number of days free of health complications, examples of positive health-promoting behavior, weight lost or hours spent in exercise). Were the outcomes that were outlined met? If not, why not? What unanticipated changes (positive and negative) resulted?

INTERVENTIONS IN PEDIATRIC ADHERENCE

Given the breadth of pediatric health concerns and types of treatment recommendations, it is beyond the scope of this chapter to discuss adherence-promoting intervention approaches comprehensively. The literature on adherence is focused largely on correlates of adherence–nonadherence, with relatively less emphasis on treatment approaches. However, sufficient empirical data are present to allow for the identification of effective intervention approaches. We present these data for their inclusion in collaborative management approaches and emphasize that they were *not* developed within a collaborative model. Thus, we are encouraging integration of these approaches into a systems-oriented treatment framework.

General Intervention Approaches to Adherence

In general, intervention approaches applied to pediatric health concerns build on well known approaches in psychology more generally (e.g., social learning, family), with tailoring to the specific needs of children with health concerns. La Greca and Schuman (1995) provide a helpful organization, highlighting interventions that emphasize: (1) learning new skills and behaviors, (2) offering supervision and/or feedback, (3) providing incentives for adherent behavior, and (4) developing family support and/or problem solving, and multicomponent interventions.

The management of a pediatric health condition requires new skills for children, families, and school personnel. Keeping pace with the rapid changes in medical treatments and technology is a challenge. At a basic level, it is unreasonable to expect adherence with medical regimens if education about the illness and treatment has not been successful. Ideally, at the point of diagnosis of an illness, or at the point of a change in illness course or treatment approach, patients and parents receive education about treatment requirements. This is often completed by nurses or other healthcare staff. Although education is helpful, it does not provide assurance that families have mastered the skills necessary to complete the regimens at home, or that potential barriers to effective compliance may not have been identified. Educational interventions may be accomplished as psychoeducation by use of modeling, or increasingly, through computer-mediated technology.

Given the importance of relationship quality and clear communication among patients, families, and staff, it is not surprising to find that a number of effective interventions for adherence focus on supervision and/or feedback related to the treatment regimens. At the simplest level, this may include regular questions and prompts from healthcare personnel regarding adherence behaviors. In the case of illnesses and treatments in which adherence can be assessed from markers in the blood, urine, or saliva (e.g., diabetes), medical monitoring tends to be more prominent. This also applies to approaches that use pill counts as outcomes in looking at adherence (e.g., ADHD, HIV).

Other approaches include visual cues or reminders (e.g., phone calls to prompt patients to take medication, keep appointments, or labeling items to increase use, such as reminder notes on the refrigerator or medicine chest). An additional intervention strategy is self-monitoring. For example, in diabetes, children may be asked to record their blood glucose levels.

As an example of the behavioral approaches used with success to increase adherence, Rapoff (1999) summarized the results of a series of single-subject studies in which token reinforcement was used to improve adherence to medication and splint wearing in children and adolescents with juvenile rheumatoid arthritis (JRA). While noting that these approaches are effective in the case of documented noncompliance, Rapoff (2000) suggested ways in which interventions for adherence could be conceptualized more broadly; that is, using a prevention model, the more intensive interventions (e.g., token reinforcement, contingency contracting, self-management, therapy) may be targeted toward patients with chronic adherence difficulties. In contrast, education, increased monitoring, and simplification of treatment protocols may be sufficiently effective and easier to implement when there is risk of adherence difficulties.

Behavioral group treatment approaches have been used with children with cystic fibrosis and their families (Stark, 2001). In this case, the adherence issue is related to the child's successful maintenance of a high-energy, high-fat diet necessitated by pancreatic insufficiency. The tested treatment protocols provide intervention for parents and patients separately, in each case emphasizing nutritional information, calorie goals, and developmentally appropriate behavioral approaches for encouraging food intake. The results of this treatment approach have been consistently strong (Stark, 2001).

Interventions that promote adherence in children with diabetes are among the most advanced in their incorporation of families into the adherence intervention models. From a family systems perspective, incorporating families in promoting adherence is essential. La Greca conducted a randomized clinical trial of a 6-week, multifamily intervention for adolescents with diabetes (with a wait-list control condition) (Satin, La Greca, Zigo, & Skyler, 1989). The intervention addressed major issues associated with adherence (e.g., communication skills, problem solving, support for self-care). The intervention also included creative elements, such as having other family members simulate the experience of having diabetes for a week in order to experience the demands of the treatment regimen. The study results were interpreted as showing the importance of family support in improving self-care outcomes.

Because adherence regimens can accentuate naturally occurring conflict in families, particularly for adolescents, interventions that address family conflict are particularly compelling. Wysocki and his colleagues (2000) have evaluated behavioral family systems therapy (BFST) in a sample of 119 families of adolescents with diabetes, comparing 10 sessions of BFST with current treatment and with an education and support condition. BFST targeted family conflict by emphasizing problem solving and negotiation, communication skills, cognitive restructuring of beliefs that may maintain conflicts, and intervening in family patterns that were contradictory to adaptive functioning. BFST was associated with improvements in family relationships and reduced diabetes-specific conflict. At the same time, however, treatment condition was not strongly associated with diabetes control and adherence. The data reflect both the advantages and disadvantages of taking a broader perspective on adherence; that is, improvements in conflict are important and may relate indirectly to variables relevant to adherence, although they may not show direct and clear relationships. BFST is currently being evaluated in another childhood chronic illness (cystic fibrosis; Quittner et al., 2001), an important step in terms of establishing commonalities in adherence treatments across diseases, as well as within illness groups.

Expanding on the notion of adolescent–parent conflict, Anderson and her team developed a brief teamwork intervention protocol to prevent the increase in conflict typically related to diabetes care over the early adolescent years (Anderson, Brackett, Ho, & Laffel, 2000). This 20–30 minute intervention is contrasted with an attention–control condition and administered by research assistants. The treatment is intriguing, because participation in the program appeared to stem the expected increase in parent–adolescent conflict seen in a comparison group. Additional research is necessary in order to determine possible indirect pathways among family variables, disease characteristics, and outcomes, including multiple measures of adherence.

Some of the most promising interventions for adherence in pediatric illness are those that include multiple intervention approaches (La Greca & Schuman, 1995). This is not surprising given the complexity of maintaining medical regimens and the many potential barriers to adherence. It is also logical, in that effective family management of complex medical routines involves a substantial degree of flexibility. By having multiple intervention approaches at hand, patients and families would ideally have more choice in using what it necessary for a particular situation. A complication of this approach is also quite evident, however. Given the current state of intervention science in adherence, we do not clearly understand what intervention approaches are most effective, when, and for whom. By combining intervention strategies into multicomponent programs, it becomes very difficult to extract the most potent components of a program, particularly because existing studies are highly variable in terms of patient groups and outcomes (Lemanek et al., 2001).

Empirically Supported Treatments

The issue of the type and strength of empirical support for adherence-related interventions warrants discussion. Although there is little argument that conducting research to show the outcomes of our intervention approaches is essential, the ways in which treatment effectiveness is measured, and whether and how guidelines for establishing effectiveness might be set, is a topic of debate within psychology now more generally. The *Journal of Pediatric Psychology* (JPP) published a series of articles on empirically support treatment (EST) in pediatric psychology in 1999–2001. The articles reviewed specific topic areas and used criteria established by a subcommittee of the Taskforce on Effective Psychosocial Interventions, based within Division 12 (Clinical Psychology) of the American Psychological Association (Chambless et al., 1996). The criteria were altered slightly for pediatric psychology interventions due to considerations such as the low incidence of pediatric illnesses and the resulting difficulties with small sample sizes (Spirito, 1999).

Treatments related to adherence for asthma, JRA, and type 1 diabetes were included in the series (Lemanek et al., 2001). In addition, pediatric obesity is addressed in a separate paper in the series (Jelalian & Saelens, 1999). These reviews used the JPP EST series criteria as follows: In order to be considered a *Well-Established* intervention, it was necessary that there be two well-conducted between-group experiments that demonstrated efficacy in one of two ways: (1) showing superiority to a pill, psychological placebo, or alternative treatment; or (2) demonstrating equivalence to an already established treatment in studies with adequate statistical power. Another way in which an intervention could be deemed *Well-Established* is if a series of nine or more well-designed, single-subject design experiments included comparison to another treatment. The studies also needed to describe the samples thoroughly, and outcomes must have been reported by two independent investigators. In the category of *Probably Efficacious*, two studies showing that the treatment was more effective than a wait-list control were required, or otherwise met somewhat relaxed criteria from the well-established interventions (e.g., may not have been replicated by two independent groups). A treatment protocol was required, although not a manual. *Promising* interventions were those for which there were positive outcomes from one well-controlled study or a small series of single-subject studies, or two or more well-controlled studies by the same investigator.

These are relatively rigorous criteria, especially considering the difficulties in conducting research in pediatric settings. In Lemanek et al.'s (2001) review, there were no adherence interventions that met criteria for a *Well-Established* treatment for the three chronic illnesses addressed. There were, however, several *Probably Efficacious* adherence interventions, including organizational strategies (e.g., changing clinic routines, simplifying treatment regimens) for asthma, behavioral approaches for JRA, and multicomponent and behavioral approaches for diabetes. With respect to childhood obesity, there are multiple reports of treatments (*Well-Established*) based on behavioral and multicomponent approaches for children and preadolescents, but not for adolescents (Jelalian & Saelens, 1999). Lemanek et al. (2001) provided thoughtful discussion points related to the conclusions of their review. Many of these issues are echoed throughout the adherence literature (e.g., definitional inconsistencies in adherence, inadequate measures of adherence). Another problem is the general lack of replication research in psychology generally. Finally, treatments that work on an individual basis (e.g., relaxation training) are readily adopted by practicing psychologists across settings. The difficulties of achieving and maintaining weight loss in adolescents highlights the potential role of collaborative management; that is, more comprehensive approaches across settings may help in addressing this difficult problem, particularly when combined with the normal developmental processes attendant to adolescence.

With regard to empirically supported treatments in a collaborative management model, we encourage the use of best practices. Those approaches that meet *Probably Efficacious* criteria will often be helpful; those that are *Promising* are certainly worth consideration. However, there are other approaches, such as those suggested throughout this chapter, related to families and systems, that have yet to be explored and subjected to scientific scrutiny. The lack of evidence for *Well-Established* treatments in adherence may be taken as encouragement for the ongoing development and evaluation of alternative approaches.

Table 5.1 summarizes some general adherence-related concerns for several pediatric conditions and examples of associated interventions for adherence. In identifying conditions for inclusion, we made no effort to be exhaustive, but rather selected a variety of conditions frequently encountered in pediatric medicine, and with a range of etiologies and treatments. As can be seen, the types of adherence problems cluster around common themes (e.g., taking medication, following dietary and exercise recommendations, and successfully accomplishing other aspects of treatment). Similarly, the types of interventions are similar across diseases and, to some extent, types of adherence concern (e.g., behavioral and family approaches). The most effective use of these intervention approaches rests on their integration into the broader collaborative management model.

CONCLUSIONS AND SUMMARY

Adherence is critically important in terms of evaluating the success of pediatric healthcare. It provides a "bottom line" in medical care; that is, effective treatments may not be effective if the treatments are not delivered successfully. Our premise throughout this chapter is that adherence is a broad construct, best framed as a process of collaborative management involving the patient, family, healthcare team, and school. We urge the development of this complex, systems-oriented model as an alternative to current frustration with the conceptualization, assessment, and intervention approaches available in the general area of adherence.

The modest empirical support for adherence interventions in pediatric healthcare, despite the general efficacy of broad approaches (e.g.,

TABLE 5.1. Adherence-Related Concerns and Interventions to Improve Adherence for Selected Pediatric Health Conditions

Pediatric health condition	Adherence-related concerns	Intervention approaches	Comments
Asthma	• Medication (bronchodilators, anti-inflamatories, inhaled and oral steroids) to manage and prevent asthma attacks • Environmental triggers avoided/controlled • Immunotherapy injections	• Educational strategies • Organizational (modifying protocol, physician monitoring) • Self-monitoring • Positive reinforcement • Multicomponent approaches	• Research is needed to identify well-established treatments.
Attention-deficit/ hyperactivity disorder (ADHD)	• Medication (stimulants) to improve attention and impulse control • Behavior therapy at home and school	• Educational strategies • Organizational (physician monitoring) • Development of interventions in partnerships with all intervention stakeholders	• Very little research has been conducted to address adherence.
Cancers	• Chemotherapy and side effects • Radiation therapy • Procedures and surgeries	• No published reports specific to treatment adherence	• Well-established treatments for pain- and chemotherapy-related distress may have indirect impact on adherence.
Cystic fibrosis	• Medication (e.g., aerosol treatment, enzyme supplements) • Diet (high-energy, high-fat diet)	• Trials underway of behavioral family systems therapy for medication adherence • Behavioral group therapy, parents/children, for diet	• Research is needed to identify well-established treatments.
Diabetes (type 1)	• Insulin injections • Diet • Exercise	• Educational strategies • Self-monitoring • Role playing/modeling • Positive reinforcement • Decision-making/problem-solving skills • Family teamwork • Behavioral family systems therapy • Multifamily groups • Multicomponent approaches	• Multicomponent and family interventions appear most effective and can target variables that may be indirectly related to adherence (e.g., family conflict).

(continued)

TABLE 5.1. (*continued*)

Pediatric health condition	Adherence-related concerns	Intervention approaches	Comments
Juvenile rheumatoid arthritis	• Medications to reduce inflammation and pain • Physical and occupational therapy for motion/strength • Surgeries, splinting	• Educational strategies • Self- and parent-monitoring • Positive reinforcement	• Research is needed to identify well-established treatments.
Obesity	• Dietary changes • Exercise	• For 8- to 12-year-olds, comprehensive behavioral interventions are effective • Parent involvement in intervention	• Need for research on treatment for adolescents.

behavioral, cognitive-behavioral, family), suggests that existing models of adherence have been too narrow in their conceptualization and scope. As an alternative, we propose a series of steps for establishing a collaborative management process that includes partnerships among families, schools, and healthcare teams. We urge the incorporation of known psychological intervention approaches (including multicomponent treatment packages) within the collaborative management approach, including readjustment of the plan as needed and evaluation of the outcomes.

REFERENCES

Anderson, B., Brackett, J., Ho, J., & Laffel, L. (2000). An intervention to promote family teamwork in diabetes management tasks: Relationships among parental involvement, adherence to blood glucose monitoring, and glycemic control in young adolescents with type 1 diabetes. In D. Drotar (Ed.), *Promoting adherence to medical treatment and chronic childhood illness: Concepts, methods and interventions* (pp. 347–366). Mahwah, NJ: Erlbaum.

Bauman, L. (2000). A patient-centered approach to adherence: Risks for nonadherence. In D. Drotar (Ed.), *Promoting adherence to medical treatment and chronic childhood illness: Concepts, methods and interventions* (pp. 71–93). Mahwah, NJ: Erlbaum.

Bell, S., & Morgan, S. (2000). Children's attitudes and behavioral intentions toward a peer presented as obese: Does a medical explanation for the obesity make a difference? *Journal of Pediatric Psychology, 25*, 137–145.

Bronfenbrenner, U. (1979). *The ecology of human development*. Cambridge, MA: Harvard University Press.

Chambless, D. L., Sanderson, W. C., Shoham, V., Bennett Johnson, S., Pope, K. S., Crits-Christoph, P., Baker, M., Johnson, B., Woody, S. R., Sue, S., Beutler, L., Williams, D. A., & McCurry, S. (1996). An update on empirically supported therapies. *Clinical Psychologist, 49,* 5–18.

Cohen, S., & Wamboldt, F. (2000). The parent–physician relationship in pediatric asthma care. *Journal of Pediatric Psychology, 25,* 69–77.

Creer, T. (2000). Self-management and the control of chronic pediatric illness. In D. Drotar (Ed.), *Promoting adherence to medical treatment and chronic childhood illness: Concepts, methods and interventions* (pp. 95–129). Mahwah, NJ: Erlbaum.

Davis, C., Delamater, A., Shaw, K., La Greca, A., Eidson, M., Perez-Rodriques, J., & Nemery, R. (2001). Brief report: Parentings styles, regimen adherence and glycemic control in 4–10 year old children with diabetes. *Journal of Pediatric Psychology, 26,* 123–129.

Drotar, D. (Ed.). (2000). *Promoting adherence to medical treatment and chronic childhood illness: Concepts, methods and interventions.* Mahwah, NJ: Erlbaum.

Fiese, B., & Wamboldt, F. (2000). Family routines, rituals and asthma management: A proposal for family-based strategies to increase treatment adherence. *Families, Systems, and Health, 18,* 405–418.

Guite, J., Walker, L., Smith, C., & Garber, J. (2000). Children's perceptions of peers with somatic symptoms: The impact of gender, stress and illness. *Journal of Pediatric Psychology, 25,* 125–135.

Haynes, R. (1979). Introduction. In R. Haynes, D. Taylor, & D. Sackett (Eds.). *Compliance in health care* (pp. 1–7). Baltimore, MD: Johns Hopkins University Press.

Horner, S. (1998). Using the Open Airways curriculum to improve self-care for third grade children with asthma. *Journal of School Health, 68,* 329–333.

Jacobson, A., Hauser, S., Lavori, P., Willett, J., Cole, C., Wolfsdorf, J., Dumont, R., & Wertlieb, D. (1994). Family environment and glycemic control: A four year prospective study of children and adolescents with insulin-dependent diabetes mellitus. *Psychosomatic Medicine, 56,* 401–409.

Jelalian, E., & Saelens, B. (1999). Empirically supported treatments in pediatric psychology: Pediatric obesity. *Journal of Pediatric Psychology, 24,* 223–248.

Johnson, B. (2000). Family-centered care: Four decades of progress. *Families, Systems, and Health, 18,* 137–156.

Kazak, A. (2001). Comprehensive care for children with cancer and their families: A social ecological framework guiding research, practice and policy. *Children's Services: Social Policy, Research and Practice, 4,* 217–233.

Kazak, A., Penati, B., Brophy, P., & Himelstein, B. (1998). Pharmacologic and psychologic interventions for procedural pan. *Pediatrics, 102,* 59–66.

Kazak, A. E., Segal-Andrews, A. M., & Johnson, K. (1995). Pediatric psychology research and practice: A family/systems approach. In M. C. Roberts (Ed.), *Handbook of pediatric psychology* (2nd ed., pp. 84–104). New York: Guilford Press.

Kazak, A., Simms, S., Barakat, L., Hobbie, W., Foley, B., Golomb, B., & Best, M. (1999). Surviving Cancer Competently Intervention Program (SCCIP): A cognitive-behavioral and family therapy intervention for adolescent suvivors of childhood cancer and their families. *Family Process, 38,* 175–192.

Kazak, A., Simms, S., & Rourke, M. (2002). Family systems practice in pediatric psychology. *Journal of Pediatric Psychology, 27,* 133–144.

Kazak, A., & Sorkin, S. (1997). Competence Encouragement Tokens (CET): Two illustrations of an innovative behavioral technique in family therapy. *Families, Systems and Health, 15,* 321–331.

Kazak, A. E., Stuber, M., Barakat, L., Meeske, K., Guthrie, D., & Meadows, A. (1998). Predicting posttraumatic stress symptoms in mothers and fathers of survivors of childhood cancer. *Journal of the American Academy of Child and Adolescent Psychiatry, 37,* 823–831.

Korsch, B., & Harding, C. (1997). *The intelligent patient's guide to the doctor–patient relationship: Learning how to talk so your doctor will listen.* New York: Oxford University Press.

La Greca, A. (1990). Issues in adherence with pediatric regimens. *Journal of Pediatric Psychology, 15,* 423–436.

La Greca, A., Prinstein, M., & Fetter, M. (2001). Adolescent peer crowd affiliation: Linkages with health-risk behaviors and close friendships. *Journal of Pediatric Psychology, 26,* 131–143.

La Greca, A., & Schuman, W. (1995). Adherence to prescribed medical regiments. In M. C. Roberts (Ed.), *Handbook of pediatric psychology* (2nd ed., pp. 55–83). New York: Guilford Press.

Lemanek, K., Kamps, J., & Chung, N. B. (2001). Empirically supported treatments in pediatric psychology: Regimen adherence. *Journal of Pediatric Psychology, 26,* 253–275.

Noll, R., LeRoy, S., Bukowski, W., Rogosch, F., & Kulkarni, R. (1991). Peer relationships and adjustment in children with cancer. *Journal of Pediatric Psychology, 16,* 307–326.

Noll, R., Vannatta, K., Koontz, K., & Kalinyak, K. (1996). Peer relationships and emotional well-being of youngsters with sickle cell disease. *Child Development, 67,* 423–436.

Persaud, D., Barnette, S., Weller, S., Baldwin, C., Niebuhr, V., & McCormick, D. (1996). An asthma self-management program for children, including instruction in peak flow monitoring by school nurses. *Journal of Asthma, 33,* 37–43.

Power, T., & Bartholomew, K. (1987). Family–school relationship patterns: An ecological perspective. *School Psychology Review, 16,* 498–512.

Power, T., Heathfield, L., McGoey, K., & Blum, N. (1999). Managing and preventing chronic health problems: School psychology's role. *School Psychology Review, 28,* 251–263.

Quittner, A., Drotar, D., Ievers-Landis, C., Slocom, N., Seidner, D., & Jacobsen, J. (2001). Adherence to medical treatments in adolescents with cystic fibrosis: The development and evaluation of family-based interventions. In D. Drotar (Ed.), *Promoting adherence to medical treatment and chronic childhood illness: Concepts, methods and interventions* (pp. 383–407). Mahwah, NJ: Erlbaum.

Rapoff, M. (1999). *Adherence to pediatric regimens.* New York: Plenum Press.

Rapoff, M. (2000). Facilitating adherence to medical regimens for pediatric rheumatic diseases: Primary, secondary and tertiary prevention. In D. Drotar (Ed.), *Promoting adherence to medical treatment and chronic childhood illness: Concepts, methods and interventions* (pp. 329–345). Mahwah, NJ: Erlbaum.

Riekert, K., & Drotar, D. (2000). Adherence to medical treatment in pediatric chronic illness: Critical issues and answered questions. In D. Drotar (Ed.), *Promoting adherence to medical treatment and chronic childhood illness: Concepts, methods and interventions* (pp. 3–32). Mahwah, NJ: Erlbaum.

Rolland, J. (1994). *Families, illness and disability: An integrative treatment model.* New York: Basic Books.

Satin, W., La Greca, A., Zigo, M., & Skyler, J. (1989). Diabetes in adolescence: Effects of multifamily group intervention and parent simulation of diabetes. *Journal of Pediatric Psychology, 14,* 259–569.

Spirito, A. (1999). Introduction. *Journal of Pediatric Psychology, 24,* 87–90.

Stark, L. (2001). Adherence to diet in chronic conditions: The example of cystic fibrosis. In D. Drotar (Ed.), *Promoting adherence to medical treatment and chronic childhood illness: Concepts, methods and interventions* (pp. 409–427). Mahwah, NJ: Erlbaum.

Sunde, E., Mabe, P., & Josephson, A. (1993). Difficult parents: From adversaries to partners. *Clinical Pediatrics, 32,* 213–219.

Tellerman, K., & Medio, F. (1993). Pediatricians' opinions of mothers. *Pediatrics, 81,* 186–189.

U.S. Department of Health and Human Services. (1999). *Mental health: A report of the Surgeon General.* Rockville, MD: U.S. Department of Health and Human Services, Center for Mental Health Services, National Institutes of Health, National Institute of Mental Health.

Wade, S., Taylor, H. G., Drotar, D., Stancin, T., & Yeates, K. (1996). Childhood traumatic brain injury: Initial impact on the family. *Journal of Learning Disabilities, 29,* 652–661.

Waters, D. (2001). Commentary: The revolutionary subtext of collaborative care. *Families, Systems and Health, 19,* 59–63.

Wysocki, T., Harris, M., Greco, P., Bubb, J., Danda, C., Harvey, L., McDonell, K., Taylor, A., & White, N. (2000). Randomized controlled trial of behavioral therapy for families of adolescents with insulin-dependent diabetes mellitus. *Journal of Pediatic Psychology, 25,* 23–33.

CHAPTER 6

Managing and Evaluating Pharmacological Interventions

Over the past several decades, the use of medication has increased exponentially in the treatment of childhood illnesses and mental disorders. In fact, pharmacotherapy has become a primary treatment for many childhood conditions. For example, approximately 6% of school-age children are treated with stimulant medication (e.g., methylphenidate) for symptoms of ADHD, with notable increases over recent years, particularly among adolescents with this disorder (Safer, Zito, & Fine, 1996). Another 6% of children under the age of 18 years suffer from asthma wherein the majority of affected individuals receive one or more medications (e.g., bronchodilators and anti-inflammatory drugs) to alleviate and/or prevent symptoms (Lemanek & Hood, 1999).

The expanded use of pharmacotherapy for treating a variety of childhood disorders has had an impact on the academic, behavioral, and social functioning of treated children in school and community settings. In some cases, medications have led to significant improvements in critical performance areas beyond intended symptom reduction effects. Methylphenidate and other psychostimulants, for example, have been found to enhance academic productivity and accuracy for many students with ADHD (Rapport, Denney, DuPaul, & Gardner, 1994). In other cases, medications have led to adverse side effects wherein functioning is deleteriously affected despite symptom reduction. For example, chemotherapy (e.g., prednisone and antineoplastics) used in treating leukemia can lead to fatigue and low energy, short-term deficits in fine-motor coordination, and, possibly, long-term diminishment in academic achievement (for review, see Handler & DuPaul, 1999).

Given that medications could affect children's performance or skills in a variety of areas, a comprehensive evaluation of medication effects *must* include measures that are sensitive to changes in academic, behavioral, and social functioning. Leaders in school, child clinical, and pediatric psychology have highlighted this need and provided models for school-based medication assessment (Barkley, Fischer, Newby, & Breen, 1988; Brown & Sawyer, 1998; Gadow, Nolan, Paolicelli, & Sprafkin, 1991; Phelps, Brown, & Power, 2002). Although these models differ to some degree with respect to specific goals, measures, and procedures, they share several critical features. First, effective medication management and evaluation involves a strong linkage and communication among family, school, and medical communities. Second, medication typically is considered and assessed in the context of other interventions, including those that address psychosocial, educational, and socioeconomic factors. The specific type and dosage of medication often is determined in relation to the potential efficacy of other treatment modalities while balancing a desire to use maximally effective, yet minimally intrusive interventions. Finally, there is an emphasis on collecting multiple measures across settings and sources to determine medication effects.

The purpose of this chapter is to discuss medication management and evaluation procedures that lie at the interface of school, family, and healthcare systems. Factors to consider when deciding whether medication is a necessary component of a child's treatment plan are reviewed. Evaluation procedures for assessing the short- and long-term effects of a medication regimen also are delineated. Although a review of the medications used with pediatric populations is beyond the scope of this chapter, two prominent examples of medications used to treat child disorders and their effects on school and community functioning are provided (including methylphenidate for ADHD and corticosteroids for pediatric asthma). More detailed information regarding specific medications for childhood disorders is available in several, recently published texts (Brown & Sawyer, 1998; Phelps et al., 2002; Werry & Aman, 1999).

DETERMINING WHETHER PHARMACOTHERAPY IS NECESSARY

Despite the fact that pharmacotherapy may be an empirically supported treatment for many pediatric disorders, this does not imply that medication is necessary in all cases or that it is sufficient to use medication in isolation. Thus, in most cases, the necessity of medication must be determined prior to initiating treatment. This is particularly important for treating behavior and emotion disorders that may be successfully impacted by nonmedical interventions. Although the specific steps in making this decision will vary across disorders and medications, a number of procedures that should be followed in all cases are discussed in detail in this section.

Comprehensive Evaluation

It is axiomatic that the first step in determining the necessity of pharmacotherapy in treating a specific disorder is a thorough diagnostic evaluation. Typically, this will require a comprehensive assessment of a child's functioning across multiple areas (e.g., physical, psychological, academic, and social), systems (e.g., medical, educational, and psychological), and settings (e.g., home, school, and community). Clearly, a detailed physical examination is a key component, because it must be determined that the child (1) exhibits prominent symptoms of the specific illness or disorder, (2) does not exhibit significant symptoms of alternative disorders that would preclude treatment with a specific medication, and (3) does not have a positive history of physical conditions that would contraindicate the use of a specific medication. In many cases, a psychological and/or psychiatric evaluation also is required to determine whether significant symptoms of behavior or emotion disorders are present, as well as to establish a baseline of functioning in cases where medications might have adverse side effects on psychosocial functioning. If there is sufficient time, an assessment of cognitive and/or academic functioning also may be necessary, particularly in those cases in which medications that could impact school performance are being considered.

Regardless of the type of evaluation being conducted, multiple sources should be consulted, especially parents, teachers, and the children themselves. Physical symptoms and problematic behaviors may vary in form, frequency, severity, and intensity across settings. Potential variation in symptoms may be missed if a single source (e.g., parents) is consulted. Consistency of symptoms is an important determinant of the need for medication. In fact, when considering stimulant medication for the treatment of ADHD, clinicians typically look for a high frequency and severity of symptoms across home and school settings (Barkley, 1998).

Response to Other Interventions

Another important determinant of the need for medication treatment is to assess a child's response to psychosocial and/or educational interventions. In many cases, particularly for children with behavior or emotion disorders, school personnel and/or community-based professionals have implemented interventions prior to consideration of pharmacotherapy. If other interventions are currently in place, one would want to assess their success and whether there is room for improvement. Several questions are important to consider:

1. Have symptoms of the disorder improved as a function of the current intervention plan?
2. Is the improvement considered sufficient by key individuals in the child's life?
3. Are any adverse side effects present that would indicate discontinuation or modification of current treatments?
4. What are the effects of the current intervention on key areas of functioning?
5. What is the likelihood that adding medication to the treatment plan will result in further, clinically significant improvement?

A number of assessment methods can be used to answer these questions. Ratings of symptoms and/or behaviors in key functioning areas (e.g., social skills) can be completed by parents, teachers, and the children themselves. Direct observations of behavior in important settings (e.g., classroom) can be conducted under intervention and nonintervention conditions. Performance measures, such as academic achievement tests or curriculum-based measurement (CBM; Shinn, 1998) probes, can be collected over a period of time. In order to address questions of social validity, consumer satisfaction ratings can be collected from key individuals. Furthermore, one can assess the social validity of treatment effects by comparing the target child's symptoms, skills, or behaviors to those exhibited by classmates or typical peers. The latter is particularly helpful when a treatment goal is normalization of child functioning. To the extent that assessment measures indicate room for improvement despite the implementation of pharmacological or psychosocial treatments, strong consideration of a combined intervention is recommended. Alternatively, in those cases in which symptoms appear to be under good control without a pharmacological or psychosocial intervention, treatment may be delayed until the child's situation warrants attention.

Decisions Based on Empirical Literature

Decisions regarding the use of pharmacotherapy for a specific disorder should be based on guidelines explicated through empirical studies. There is a growing literature supporting the use of medication for the treatment of a variety of childhood disorders, ranging from chronic illnesses to emotion and behavior disorders (for review, see Phelps et al., 2002; Werry & Aman, 1999). In recent years, a number of comprehensive reviews of the literature that have been published are supportive of pharmacotherapy for asthma (Lemanek, Trane, & Weiner, 1999), ADHD (Spencer, Biederman, Wilens, Harding, O'Donnell, & Griffin, 1996), enuresis (Houts, Berman, & Abramson, 1994), obsessive–compulsive disorder (Scahill, 1996), anxiety disorders (March, 1999), tic disorders (Castellanos, 1998), and pain (Bursch, Walco, & Zeltzer, 1998). Extant studies provide important information regarding the behavior and symptoms most likely to be affected by a given medication, as well as the dosage range that is safe and effective for the treatment of specific disorders. The research literature also can provide information on the limitations of pharmacotherapy for the treatment of certain disorders, such as autism and developmental disabilities (Volkmar, 2001).

Typically, literature reviews provide a description of studies and their outcomes, as well as interpretations and guidelines based on these descriptions. Of greater value are reviews that include quantitative analyses of the literature (i.e., meta-analyses). Meta-analyses involve the calculation of effect sizes that take into account mean differences between treatment and control groups, while accounting for expected between-subject variation in the absence of treatment (see Hedges & Olkin, 1985; Rosenthal, 1984). Thus, medication effects are quantified in terms of standard deviation units wherein effect sizes of 0.2, 0.5, and 0.8 are considered small, medium, and large, respectively (Cohen, 1992). Unfortunately, few meta-analyses have been included in the medication literature. As an example, Kavale (1982) found relatively large effect sizes (i.e., 0.80) for stimulant medications used to treat ADHD.

Empirical studies provide important information regarding the magnitude and dose-related nature of medication effects at a group level and can therefore provide guidance at a general level as to whether a specific medication and dose range will be helpful for an individual child. It should be noted, however, that medication response varies considerably across individual children as a function of body weight, age, or physiological functioning. Ultimately, decisions about medication effects must be made at the individual level and should be based on data collected regarding changes in symptoms, behaviors, and/or other aspects of functioning (see the following Medication Evaluation Procedures section).

Collaborative Decision Making

The American Academy of Pediatrics (AAP; 2001) has recommended that decisions regarding the use and effects of medication be made through discussion and collaboration among a child's parents, physician, psychologist, educators, and other involved professionals. Team decision making allows for the consideration of alternate treatment options and for cooperation in evaluating medication effects. Although physicians are in the best position to delineate specific medication options, it is clear that environmental, psychological, educational, and social factors are important to consider both prior to and following pharmacotherapy.

Examples of a collaborative approach to medication decision making are provided in the recent guidelines for prescribing stimulant medication, published by the American Academy of Child and Adolescent Psychiatry (AACAP; 2002), and for the treatment of ADHD, published by the AAP (2001). One of the primary recommendations of the latter report is that the treating physician, the parents, and the child should collaborate with school personnel in determining appropriate targets for treatment. Furthermore, parental and child acceptability of the potential pharmacotherapy regimen should be assessed prior to conducting a medication trial. In particular, whether the parents perceive the need for medication and understand the potential effects and side effects of drug therapy should be assessed. These perceptions have an impact on how healthcare professionals explain the need for pharmacotherapy, as well as the decision to prescribe medication as a first-line treatment. For example, parents tend to view pharmacotherapy less favorably than psychosocial interventions for disruptive behavior disorders such as ADHD (Liu, Robin, Brenner, & Eastman, 1991). Thus, physicians should explain clearly why medication is necessary (e.g., due to severity of symptoms), what symptoms will and will not be addressed by this treatment, what side effects are possible, as well as how side effects will be addressed when they arise. There may be times when parents are so resistant to medication that alternative treatments are attempted first and pharmacotherapy is postponed, at least until initial treatment response is determined.

Another key recommendation from the AACAP and AAP guidelines is for prescribing clinicians to monitor medication effects periodically by obtaining specific information from parents, teachers, and children. Ultimately, final decisions regarding the ongoing use of medication are made by the child's parents and physician, because they have the primary responsibility for the child's welfare. However, it is clear that ongoing communication among treatment team members will be necessary to determine the optimal dosage of medication and thereby enhance the overall treatment plan.

MEDICATION EVALUATION PROCEDURES

A data-based evaluation process must be used to ensure that prescribed medications elicit the desired effect, while minimizing unwanted, adverse side effects. A number of medication evaluation models have been proposed, particularly for the assessment of stimulant medication effects on the behavior of children with ADHD (e.g., Barkley et al., 1988; Gadow et al., 1991; Rapport et al., 1994). In addition, a number of texts have delineated medication monitoring procedures that might be used beyond the stimulant class (e.g., Brown & Sawyer, 1998; Phelps et al., 2002). The various medication evaluation models have included a number of important common features, as listed in Table 6.1. Each of these features is discussed here in the context of describing a process for examining medication effects, particularly within school settings.

Initial Evaluation of Medication Effects

Once a decision has been made to prescribe a specific medication for a child's disorder, a medication trial should be set up by the physician, parents, psychologist, and other related treatment team members. First, the team determines the time period over which the medication trial should be conducted. For some short-acting medications (e.g., methylphenidate), the evaluation can take place over a period of days or weeks. Alternatively, some medications require gradual titration (e.g., haloperidol), thereby necessitating an evaluation over the course of several weeks or months.

Next, the team needs to identify the specific areas of functioning that should be assessed in the course of the trial. Typically, the most important areas to assess will include physical, social, behavioral–emotional, and academic functioning. Decisions as to which areas to assess

---

TABLE 6.1. Important Features of Medication Evaluation Procedures

1. Medication trial designed through consultation between school- or clinic-based team and the prescribing physician.

2. Specific time lines, measures, and procedures are identified and agreed upon.

3. Areas of functioning (e.g., cognitive, academic, and behavioral) to assess are identified, and measures to assess these are utilized.

4. Objective, psychometrically sound measures (e.g., behavior rating scales and direct observations) are highly desirable.

5. Potential side effects are identified and measures to assess these are utilized.

6. Data are collected during both nonmedication and medication conditions in as controlled a fashion as possible.

7. Data are summarized through graphic display and/or tabular presentation of statistics to facilitate interpretation.

8. Interpretation of outcomes is made collaboratively with the child's physician, and recommendations are clearly communicated to the child's parents.

will be based on (1) the nature and severity of the child's disorder, (2) areas of functioning likely to be affected by medication (either in a positive or adverse manner), (3) the child's age and level of development, and (4) the feasibility of collecting data in a specific area.

Once the areas to assess are determined, specific measures and methods need to be identified to evaluate functioning. Measures might include tests of physiological functioning and physical symptoms, behavior rating scales, direct observations of behavior, brief probes of academic functioning, and self-report indices (for more details regarding assessment measures, see Brown & Sawyer, 1998; Phelps et al., 2002). Assessment measures should be psychometrically sound (i.e., possess adequate levels of reliability and validity), be brief enough to be administered on a frequent basis, and have established sensitivity to medication effects.

After delineating the specific medication, evaluation time line, and assessment procedures to be used, the team needs to outline the medication evaluation procedures. Specific dosages and their sequence need to be determined. Ideally, the dosage sequence is randomly determined, and assessment is conducted under double-blind, placebo-controlled conditions. This methodology, although ideal, can be cumbersome and impractical in many situations; however, the aim would be to approximate double-blind procedures as closely as possible. At a minimum, data should be collected during a nonmedication condition (e.g., period of time prior to initiation of medication treatment). The teacher could be kept blind to dosage by having the child take the medication in the nurse's office.

The team also needs to determine when and how frequently specific assessment measures will be collected. Frequency of collection may vary across measures, with some (e.g., behavior rating scales) administered on a weekly basis, whereas others (e.g., CBM probes) are collected more often (e.g., twice per week). CBM involves brief (1- to 2-minute) probes of academic skills that are derived directly from the child's classroom curriculum (Shinn, 1998). As such, this measure lends itself to frequent collection wherein the trajectory of skills acquisition can be documented during both treatment and nontreatment conditions. Finally, responsibilities for collecting medication trial data need to be assigned and agreed upon by team members. Typically, parents, teachers, and/or children are asked to complete one or more questionnaires on a weekly or monthly basis; the school psychologist, counselor, or special educator collects direct observation data in the classroom and/or playground; the physician and/or nurse assesses physical functioning; and the teacher, school psychologist, or special educator collects academic performance data.

In addition to collecting data on symptoms and behaviors that may be improved by the medication, the evaluation needs to include assessment of potential, adverse side effects. In particular, the team needs to consider whether a particular medication is likely to have iatrogenic effects on key aspects of school functioning, including cognitive, social, and/or academic skills. A popular method to detect side effects is to ask teachers, parents, or children about the frequency and/or severity of physical symptoms, behaviors, emotions, or cognitions that have been found associated with a specific medication in prior cases. For example, Barkley (1991) developed a brief rating scale for evaluating possible side effects of stimulant medication that has been used for both clinical and research purposes. It is important to note that the side-effect profile in a specific case may differ depending on who is asked to report it. DuPaul, Anastopoulos, Kwasnik, Barkley, and McMurray (1996) found that children reported more severe side effects of methylphenidate (relative to placebo conditions) than did parents or teachers. The ideal strategy would be to obtain side-effects ratings from parents, teachers, *and* children, although this is not feasible in all cases. In the case of potential adverse effects on academic or cognitive functioning, assessment measures might include brief cognitive tests, academic achievement tests, CBM probes, or permanent products reflecting these domains (e.g., classwork completed by the child). Furthermore, side effects need to be assessed during medication and nonmedication conditions, because behaviors or symptoms that might be interpreted as "side effects" may, in some cases, be present prior to treatment.

Once the medication evaluation has been completed, the team is responsible for summarizing and interpreting the outcome data. Data for each critical measure should be displayed in tabular or graphic format, so that the clinician can view potential treatment-induced changes across dosage conditions (including nonmedication and/or placebo phases). Ideally, interpretation of outcomes is facilitated by using analytic methods, typically employed in single-subject research designs (DuPaul & Barkley, 1993; Kazdin, 1982). Specifically, changes in level, trend, intercept, and variability can be discerned. For example, Northup and colleagues (1997, 1999) have conducted several studies using single-subject analyses to determine methylphenidate effects on the classroom performance of children with ADHD. It should be noted that single-subject analyses require multiple data points per phase that may be available for some measures (e.g., direct observations and CBM probes) and not others (e.g., behavior rating scales).

Even for measures in which one data point per medication phase is available, there are methods for determining whether medication effects might be present. For example, the reliable change index (Jacobsen & Truax, 1991) has been used to determine whether the behavior of children with ADHD has been significantly improved by methylphenidate beyond placebo-control levels (e.g., Rapport et al., 1994). The reliable change index takes into account the standard error of measurement of the specific assessment device and, as such, indicates when differences in scores across conditions are not readily accounted for by the reliability of the instrument and regression to the mean artifacts. The use of the reliable change index and similar formulas requires measures that have known psychometric properties.

Based on the data analysis conducted by the team, three questions must be answered. First, do any of the active medication conditions lead to reliable change in the desired direction? Stated differently, is there any evidence for a medication effect? If any single medication condition leads to reliable change for a specific measure relative to baseline or nonmedication phases, then an overall medication effect appears to be present.

The second question related to the data analysis is what is the lowest dose that leads to the greatest change with the least side effects? This has been referred to as identifying the minimally effective dose (Gadow, 1986). The team first determines which dosage conditions led to reliable change in the therapeutic direction. Then, those dosages that did not increase the frequency and/or severity of potential side effects relative to placebo or control conditions are highlighted. Finally, the lowest dosage among those remaining is identified.

After the minimally effective dose is determined for each of the key outcome measures, the final question for the team to consider is whether there are consistent results across assessment indices. To what degree is there consistency in dose–response across symptoms, behaviors, and/or test results? Of course, the ideal scenario would be for the same minimally effective dose to be identified across all critical measures. Unfortunately, this degree of consistency is rarely encountered in typical clinical circumstances. Thus, in most cases, the team has to determine the dosage that either (1) is identified *most frequently* as the minimally effective dosage or (2) is the minimally effective dosage for *one or more of the most critical outcomes*. For example, the dosage of albuterol that leads to the best pulmonary functioning based on peak flow readings with minimal side effects might be identified as optimal regardless of its effects on less important outcomes.

After the evaluation team has reached a conclusion as to overall medication effects and has a recommendation regarding dosage, these findings can be communicated to the family and prescribing physician (if they have not been involved on an ongoing basis in the evaluation process). The form and content of communication with families and physicians typically will differ. The most effective way to communicate medication evaluation results to physicians will be in the form of a brief written report, with a graphic summary of data included as an appendix (Drotar, 1995; DuPaul & Stoner, 2003). Given the time constraints faced by most physicians, this report should be concise, to the point, and should clearly highlight the reasons why a particular medication or dosage is being supported by the outcome data. Because physicians may not be familiar with assessment measures used by psychologists and educators, all tests, observations, and similar indices should be described in everyday terms. Often, it is helpful to follow a written report with a phone call to the physician, to briefly summarize key aspects of the medication evaluation, answer questions, and clear up any misunderstandings.

Although families also should be provided with written and oral feedback regarding the medication evaluation outcome, we recommend that communication with parents should occur in reverse order of that recommended for physicians. The team meets with parents and, possibly, the child, to explain what results were obtained and what these data indicate. Assessment measures and their results are described in layperson's terms. Showing families the results using data graphs can be particularly helpful, especially if these are explained in a clear, jargon-free manner. Furthermore, it is important for the team to recognize that parents may have concerns about the ongoing use of medication. The need for periodic reevaluation of medication response is emphasized and explained. Finally, the family is provided with a copy of the written report that was sent to the physician. It might be helpful to attach a glossary or other explanatory device to the written report, so that it is as understandable as possible.

Monitoring Long-Term Effects of Medication

Many childhood disorders are chronic and, therefore, require pharmacotherapy over extended periods of time. Adjustments in either the specific type or dosage of medication may be needed as children mature physically, emotionally, and behaviorally. Possible changes in medication are best made in the context of objective data. Thus, the medication evaluation team may periodically conduct reevaluations of treatment response. Although a reevaluation typically will be more streamlined and less comprehensive in scope than an initial evaluation, the same factors and questions need to be considered.

The frequency with which reevaluations are conducted can be determined at the conclusion of the initial medication evaluation. Some medications will require monthly or semiannual reassessments, but others may be evaluated less frequently, such as once per year. If possible, each reevaluation should include at least two conditions: (1) the current dosage and (1) a nonmedication control. In some cases, the physician and family may want to explore the effects of alternate dosages or even different medications, thereby requiring additional assessment conditions.

Specific areas of functioning that require ongoing assessment will need to be delineated. In particular, medication effects on cognition, behavior, and/or academic achievement should be assessed for those compounds that could impact these important areas. Keystone measures used during the initial evaluation may be chosen for this purpose.

As was the case for the initial evaluation, outcome data can be graphically displayed and analyzed using single-subject design methods or the reliable change index. These results may point to one of several recommendations: (1) Continue with present medication regimen; (2) keep the same medication but change dosage; (3) change the medication; or (4) discontinue pharmacotherapy. It is important for the team to consider possible psychosocial and/or educational interventions that could either replace or supplement pharmacotherapy. Periodic reevaluations are ideal opportunities for alternative treatments to be considered and possibly assessed relative to current medication conditions.

Adjustments to chronic pharmacotherapy are facilitated not only by conducting periodic reevaluations but also by maintaining ongoing communication with the prescribing physician and the family. The nature of this communication can range from informal, periodic phone calls to more formal written reports. The latter will be necessary following each structured reevaluation, and communication strategies outlined earlier for the initial evaluation should be followed.

Practical Limitations of School- and Community-Based Medication Evaluations

Implementation of the medication evaluation recommendations, stated earlier, in nonacademic settings (e.g., schools, clinics, and hospitals) can be limited by several factors. First, it may not be possible to collect data across multiple measures on a relatively continuous basis, because team members may not have the time available to do so. School-based and healthcare professionals often have multiple responsibilities that may preclude devoting much time to any individual case. Second, there may be resource constraints that could limit the comprehensiveness of a medication evaluation. For example, due to inadequate school funding, certain personnel (e.g., school nurse) may be unavailable, thereby limiting the potential assessment activities of the evaluation team. In healthcare settings, managed care and other cost-reduction factors could significantly hamper medication evaluation efforts due to lack of available personnel. Furthermore, some health insurance plans may not provide adequate compensation for medication assessment, thereby constraining these activities. Finally, medication evaluation procedures may be limited by the specific properties of the drug being assessed. For example, some medications (e.g., bupropion) may require titration over days or weeks wherein dosage changes require extensive time. Therefore, assessment becomes complicated by decisions as to when to collect data during the titration period. Furthermore, parents and teachers may not tolerate a medication evaluation that extends across weeks and, possibly, months.

Given these potential limitations, decisions must be made a priori as to adjustments in the content and process of the medication evaluation. Stated differently, the evaluation team must balance the need for an objective, comprehensive assessment on the one hand, and the need to conduct an assessment that is practically feasible and ultimately will be completed on the other. This may require tailoring the evaluation protocol to include fewer measures or less frequent assessment. The most common example of a "real-world" modification to medication evaluation protocols is the replacement of a placebo control with a no-medication condition. Although the latter does not control for expectancy or nonspecific effects of pharmacotherapy, a no-medication condition typically is more feasible and provides a baseline against which to measure drug effects. The overall objective, then, is to identify those data and procedures that will provide the best information possible in order to make objective medication decisions, while not compromising a child's safety or the time and resource limits of the setting.

CASE ILLUSTRATIONS OF MEDICATION MONITORING
Physical Health Problem

Juanita, an 11-year-old, fifth-grade student, attended a large, urban elementary school. Although Spanish was the primary language spoken at home, Juanita was fluent in both Spanish and English. She was placed in a general education classroom for all academic subjects but was receiving special education resource room help in reading several times per week. She was diagnosed with mild, intermittent asthma when she was 5 years old, but this condition did not require chronic administration of medication. Recently, her symptoms had increased in frequency and severity, to the point that she had missed several days of school. Thus, her physician and parents had decided to initiate a brief trial of an oral corticosteroid. Because this involved medication administration at school, and also because of the potential effects of this drug on Juanita's mood and cognitive functioning (see Bender, 1999), the school nurse was contacted by Juanita's physician.

Several assessment measures were collected across pre- and post-medication conditions. The school nurse agreed to collect peak flow meter readings (i.e., representing pulmonary functioning) each day at lunchtime over several weeks. In addition, Juanita's reading and math teachers collected samples of her schoolwork throughout this time period to gauge any changes in the quantity or quality of her work. On two occasions (i.e., prior to beginning corticosteroids and 2 weeks after treatment had been implemented), these teachers also provided ratings of Juanita's mood and behavior using items selected from the Teacher Report Form of the Child Behavior Checklist (Achenbach, 1991). Juanita also completed two brief rating scales at the same time points: the Children's Depression Inventory (Kovacs, 1985) and the Revised Children's Manifest Anxiety Scale (Reynolds & Paget, 1983) to provide self-report data regarding possible mood change. Because Juanita's parents were unable to read English, they were not asked to complete rating scales; however, the school nurse did interview them briefly about possible changes in Juanita's breathing and mood after medication was prescribed.

The results of this evaluation indicated that Juanita's peak flow performance was notably improved with systemic corticosteroid treatment. During nonmedication conditions, the mean peak flow was 110 liters/minute, whereas active treatment readings averaged 180 liters/minute. This represented a change from the "yellow" (or moderately impaired) zone to the "green" (or normal functioning) zone. Neither Juanita nor her teachers reported any significant changes in her emotional or behavioral functioning, nor was there any apparent impact on the quality of her school work. The use of the corticosteroid was discontinued, and the outcome data indicated that this treatment was a viable treatment if moderate to severe asthmatic symptoms reemerged in the future.

Mental Health Problem

Barry, a 7-year-old, second-grade student, was placed in a general education classroom in a moderately sized, suburban elementary school. He had been diagnosed with ADHD, combined type, by a child psychiatrist using DSM-IV (American Psychiatric Association, 1994) criteria. Although classroom- and home-based behavior modification systems had been implemented with a moderate degree of success, Barry continued to exhibit significant problems with timely and accurate work completion and consistent following of classroom rules. Therefore, his physician, parents, teachers, school psychologist, and school nurse decided to evaluate Barry's response to several dosages of AdderallXR, a psycho-stimulant medication found to be effective in reducing ADHD symptoms (Pelham et al., 2000).

The team decided to conduct an assessment across a 4-week period, wherein Barry received a different dosage of AdderallXR each week. Assessment conditions included no medication, 5 mg, 10 mg, and 15 mg. Medication was administered once per day (prior to leaving home for school), because this drug has a longer time course than other drugs (e.g., methylphenidate) that typically are administered twice per day. The order of the dosages was randomly determined, and Barry still went to the school nurse on a daily basis during the no-medication condition (and received a vitamin), thereby helping to keep the teacher blind to the dosage conditions. Assessment measures included weekly parent and teacher ratings on the ADHD Rating Scale–IV (DuPaul, Power, Anastopoulos, & Reid, 1998) and a side-effect rating scale (Barkley, 1991). The school psychologist observed Barry's on-task behavior and activity level two or three times per week during a 20-minute independent seatwork period in his regular classroom. Barry's teacher collected samples of his school work, so that the team could assess possible improvements in the completion and accuracy of his work.

As displayed in Figure 6.1, Barry showed notable improvement in the completion and accuracy of his work during the 10- and 15-mg conditions relative to the no-medication condition. Side effects were minimal for the 10-mg dosage and included slight appetite reduction and some mild insomnia. The team recommended to his physician that Barry continue to receive AdderallXR 10 mg on a regular basis, with periodic evaluation of blood pressure and physical growth. They also provided suggestions to Barry's parents to help address his mild appetite and sleep difficulties (e.g., preparing a meal for him later in the evening, when his appetite returned).

CONCLUSIONS

Given the increased use of pharmacotherapy to treat a variety of childhood disorders, it is critical for child psychologists to understand the impact of medications on social, cognitive, and behavioral functioning of children. Furthermore, psychologists must collaborate with physicians, parents, teachers, and children to determine (1) whether medication is necessary for a given condition, (2) what medication and dosage are most effective, and (3) whether periodic adjustments in dosage or type of medication are required when this treatment is used on a chronic basis. We have described a generic process for addressing these issues in school

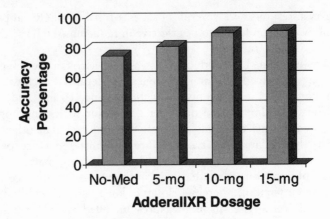

FIGURE 6.1. Percentage of school work completed accurately by a 7-year-old boy treated with several dosages of AdderallXR for ADHD.

settings. Although empirically supported procedures are available for monitoring some specific medications (e.g., stimulants for treating ADHD), research is sorely needed to delineate reliable and valid ways to assess the effects of other drugs commonly used to treat childhood disorders. Pediatric, school, and clinical child psychologists possess the necessary research and assessment training to contribute to these research efforts.

REFERENCES

Achenbach, T. M. (1991). *Teacher Report Form of the Child Behavior Checklist.* Burlington, VT: Author.

American Academy of Child and Adolescent Psychiatry. (2002). Practice parameters for the use of stimulant medications in the treatment of children, adolescents, and adults. *Journal of the American Academy of Child and Adolescent Psychiatry, 41*(Suppl. 2), 26S–49S.

American Academy of Pediatrics. (2001). Clinical practice guideline: Treatment of the school-aged child with attention-deficit/hyperactivity disorder. *Pediatrics, 108,* 1033–1044.

American Psychiatric Association. (1994). *Diagnostic and statistical manual of mental disorders* (4th ed.). Washington, DC: Author.

Barkley, R. A. (1991). *Attention-deficit hyperactivity disorder: A clinical workbook.* New York: Guilford Press.

Barkley, R. A. (1998). *Attention-deficit hyperactivity disorder: A handbook for diagnosis and treatment* (2nd ed.). New York: Guilford Press.

Barkley, R. A., Fischer, M., Newby, R. F., & Breen, M. J. (1988). Development of a multimethod clinical protocol for assessing stimulant drug responses in children with attention deficit disorder. *Journal of Clinical Child Psychology, 17,* 14–24.

Bender, B. C. (1999). Learning disorders associated with asthma and allergies. *School Psychology Review, 28,* 204–214.

Brown, R. T., & Sawyer, M. G. (1998). *Medications for school-age children: Effects on learning and behavior.* New York: Guilford Press.

Bursch, B., Walco, G. A., & Zeltzer, L. (1998). Clinical assessment and management of chronic pain and pain-associated disability syndrome. *Developmental and Behavioral Pediatrics, 19,* 45–53.

Castellanos, F. X. (1998). Tic disorders and obsessive–compulsive disorder. In B. T. Walsh (Ed.), *Child psychopharmacology* (pp. 1–28). Washington, DC: American Psychiatric Press.

Cohen, J. (1992). A power primer. *Psychological Bulletin, 112,* 155–169.

Drotar, D. (1995). *Consulting with pediatricians: Psychological perspectives.* New York: Plenum Press.

DuPaul, G. J., Anastopoulos, A. D., Kwasnik, D., Barkley, R. A., & McMurray, M. B. (1996). Methylphenidate effects on children with attention deficit hyperactivity disorder: Self-report of symptoms, side-effects, and self-esteem. *Journal of Attention Disorders, 1,* 3–15.

DuPaul, G. J., & Barkley, R. A. (1993). Behavioral contributions to pharmacotherapy: The utility of behavioral methodology in medication treatment of children with attention deficit hyperactivity disorder. *Behavior Therapy, 24,* 47–65.

DuPaul, G. J., Power, T. J., Anastopoulos, A. D., & Reid, R. (1998). *ADHD Rating Scale–IV: Checklists, norms, and clinical interpretation.* New York: Guilford Press.

DuPaul, G. J., & Stoner, G. (2003). *ADHD in the schools: Assessment and intervention strategies* (2nd Ed.). New York: Guilford Press.

Gadow, K. D. (1986). *Children on medication: Vol. 1. Hyperactivity, learning disabilities, and mental retardation.* San Diego: College-Hill Press.

Gadow, K. D., Nolan, E. E., Paolicelli, L. M., & Sprafkin, J. (1991). A procedure for assessing the effects of methylphenidate on hyperactive children in public school settings. *Journal of Clinical Child Psychology, 20,* 268–276.

Greenhill, L. L., & Osman, B. B. (Eds.) (2000). *Ritalin: Theory and practice* (2nd ed.). Larchmont, NY: Mary Ann Liebert.

Handler, M. W., & DuPaul, G. J. (1999). Pharmacological issues and iatrogenic effects on learning. In R. T. Brown (Ed.), *Cognitive aspects of chronic illness in children* (pp. 355–385). New York: Guilford Press.

Hedges, L. V., & Olkin, I. (1985). *Statistical methods for meta-analysis.* New York: Academic Press.

Houts, A. C., Berman, J. S., & Abramson, H. (1994). Effectiveness of psychological and pharmacological treatments for nocturnal enuresis. *Journal of Consulting and Clinical Psychology, 62,* 737–745.

Jacobsen, N. S., & Truax, P. (1991). Clinical significance: A statistical approach to defining meaningful change in psychotherapy research. *Journal of Consulting and Clinical Psychology, 59,* 12–19.

Kavale, K. (1982). The efficacy of stimulant drug treatment for hyperactivity: A meta-analysis. *Journal of Learning Disabilities, 15,* 280–289.

Kazdin, A. E. (1982). *Single-case research designs: Methods for clinical and applied settings.* New York: Oxford University Press.

Kovacs, M. (1985). The Children's Depression Inventory (CDI). *Psychopharmacology Bulletin, 21,* 995–998.

Lemanek, K. L., & Hood, C. (1999). Asthma. In R. T. Brown (Ed.), *Cognitive aspects of chronic illness in children* (pp. 78–104). New York: Guilford Press.

Lemanek, K. L., Trane, S. T., & Weiner, R. E. (1999). Asthma. In A. Goreczny & M. Hersen (Eds.), *Handbook of pediatric and adolescent health psychology* (pp. 141–158). Needham Heights, MA: Allyn & Bacon.

Liu, C., Robin, A. L., Brenner, S., & Eastman, J. (1991). Social acceptability of methylphenidate and behavior modification for treating attention deficit hyperactivity disorder. *Pediatrics, 88,* 560–565.

March, J. (1999). Pharmacotherapy of pediatric anxiety disorders: A critical review. In D. Beidel (Ed.), *Treating anxiety disorders in youth: Current problems and future solutions* (pp. 42–62). Washington, DC: Anxiety Disorders Association of America.

Northup, J., Fusilier, I., Swanson, V., Huete, J., Bruce, T., Freeland, J., Gulley, V., & Edwards, S. (1999). Further analysis of the separate and interactive effects of methylphenidate and common classroom contingencies. *Journal of Applied Behavior Analysis, 32,* 35–50.

Northup, J., Jones, K., Broussard, C., DiGiovanni, G., Herring, M., Fusilier, I., & Hanchey, A. (1997). A preliminary analysis of interactive effects between common classroom contingencies and methylphenidate. *Journal of Applied Behavior Analysis, 30,* 121–125.

Pelham, W. E., Gnagy, E. M., Greiner, A. R., Hoza, B., Hinshaw, S. P., Swanson, J. M., Simpson, S., Shapiro, C., Bukstein, O., Baron-Myak, C., & McBurnett, K. (2000). Behavioral versus behavioral and pharmacological treatment in ADHD children attending a summer camp program. *Journal of Abnormal Child Psychology, 28,* 507–525.

Phelps, L., Brown, R. T., & Power, T. J. (2002). *Pediatric psychopharmacology: Combining medical and psychosocial interventions.* Washington, DC: American Psychological Association.

Rapport, M. D., Denney, C., DuPaul, G. J., & Gardner, M. J. (1994). Attention deficit disorder and methylphenidate: Normalization rates, clinical effectiveness, and response prediction in 76 children. *Journal of the American Academy of Child and Adolescent Psychiatry, 33,* 882–893.

Reynolds, C. R., & Paget, K. D. (1983). National normative and reliability data for the Revised Children's Manifest Anxiety Scale. *School Psychology Review, 12,* 324–336.

Rosenthal, R. (1984). *Meta-analytic procedures for social research.* Beverly Hills, CA: Sage.

Safer, D., Zito, J., & Fine, E. (1996). Increased methylphenidate usage for attention deficit hyperactivity disorder in the 1990's. *Pediatrics, 98,* 1084–1088.

Scahill, L. (1996). Contemporary approaches to pharmacotherapy in Tourette's syndrome and obsessive–compulsive disorder. *Journal of Child and Adolescent Psychiatric Nursing, 9,* 27–44.

Shinn, M. R. (Ed.). (1998). *Advanced applications of curriculum-based measurement.* New York: Guilford Press.

Spencer, T., Biederman, J., Wilens, T., Harding, M., O'Donnell, D., & Griffin, S. (1996). Pharmacotherapy of attention-deficit hyperactivity disorder across the life cycle. *Journal of the American Academy of Child and Adolescent Psychiatry, 35,* 409–432.

Volkmar, F. R. (2001). Pharmacological interventions in autism: Theoretical and practical issues. *Journal of Clinical Child Psychology, 30,* 80–87.

Werry, J. S., & Aman, M. G. (Eds.). (1999). *Practitioner's guide to psychoactive drugs for children and adolescents* (2nd ed). New York: Plenum Press.

PART III

Developing Prevention Strategies

CHAPTER 7

Developing Selective and Indicated Prevention Programs

In recent years, there has been a change in the terminology used to refer to prevention programs. For many decades, prevention programs were designated as primary, secondary, and tertiary (Caplan, 1964). Primary prevention refers to efforts focused at the general population to prevent the occurrence of problems. Secondary prevention refers to initiatives targeted for individuals demonstrating evidence of emerging problems or signs of risk, for the purpose of impeding the development of serious difficulties. Tertiary prevention refers to efforts to intervene on behalf of individuals with identified problems, to reduce the impact of the problems and prevent the occurrence of even more serious difficulties.

One of the concerns with this terminology is that it fails to distinguish clearly tertiary prevention and intervention (Durlak, 1997). Another problem is that it does not differentiate prevention programs targeted for all children from those focused on a subgroup of healthy children who may be at risk for problems in health and development by virtue of known risk factors, such as low income status, single parents, and, in some instances, ethnic minority status (Natriello, McDill, & Pallas, 1990; Wilson, Rodrique, & Taylor, 1997).

The new terminology for prevention helps to clarify some important distinctions among types of prevention by differentiating programs into three types: universal, selective, and indicated (Institute of Medicine, 1994). Distinctions among these types of prevention are outlined in Table 7.1. Universal prevention refers to efforts to promote healthy development and to prevent the occurrence of problems targeted for all children in the general population, including those who are in high-risk

TABLE 7.1. Distinctions among Types of Prevention Programs for Children

Type	Purpose	Target group
Universal	Promote health; prevent risk.	All children in general population.
Selective	Prevent risk.	Subset of children in general population at heightened risk for disease or disorder.
Indicated	Reduce risk or impact of risk.	Children identified as having one or more risk factors related to a disease or disorder.

groups and those who are not. For example, programs to promote healthy eating and exercise habits for all children to prevent the occurrence of cardiovascular problems are examples of universal prevention initiatives (Williams et al., 1998). Another example of universal prevention is an immunization program to prevent diseases such as measles and polio (Peterson & Oliver, 1995). Universal prevention programs generally are targeted for large groups of individuals at a national, state, or local level.

Selective prevention refers to initiatives to prevent the emergence of problems among subgroups known to be at heightened risk for unhealthy patterns of behavior. For example, children who are coping with the divorce of their parents are known to be at risk for emotional, behavioral, and health problems (Wallerstein, 1987). Programs have been developed to address the emotional needs of these youngsters to prevent the emergence of health problems (Pedro-Carroll & Cowen, 1985). Similarly, preschoolers from low-income families are known to be at risk for poor educational and health outcomes (Ramey & Ramey, 1998). The Head Start program was established in the 1960s to address the needs of these children and their families, to promote the development of cognitive and social skills and to prevent the emergence of health problems later in life (Zigler & Muenchow, 1992).

Indicated prevention refers to initiatives targeted for individuals with emerging problems or signs of risk and is designed to reduce the impact of risk and to prevent the development of serious difficulties. For example, many empirically supported prevention programs have been designed for children who demonstrate evidence of aggressive behavior, in order to prevent the emergence of antisocial patterns and the occurrence of violent actions (see Greenberg, Domitrovitch, & Bumbarger, 2001; Leff, Power, Manz, Costigan, & Nabors, 2001). Similarly, programs have been developed for children with high cholesterol and/or obesity in order to prevent the emergence of cardiovascular disease (e.g., Harrell et al., 1998).

This chapter focuses on the development of selective and indicated programs of prevention (see Chapter 8 for a description of universal prevention programs). The purpose of this chapter is to (1) describe a developmental–ecological model for developing selective and indicated prevention programs, (2) outline key components in developing socially valid, culturally responsive prevention programs, and (3) provide a summary of model programs for preventing health and mental health problems. This chapter addresses prevention issues related to children who are healthy or at risk for health problems. In contrast, a prevention framework applied to children who have identified health conditions but are healthy or at risk from a mental health perspective is described in Chapter 2.

A DEVELOPMENTAL–ECOLOGICAL MODEL OF PREVENTION

The science and practice of prevention has been strongly influenced by research in developmental psychology related to psychopathology and resilience (Cicchetti & Toth, 1998; Loeber & Hay, 1997; Masten & Coatsworth, 1998). This large body of research has affirmed that health problems and psychopathology have multiple determinants, including biological and psychological factors related to the child, as well as ecological factors related to the systems in which individuals function. Health outcomes emerge as a complex transaction of individual and systemic factors over an extended period of time (Sameroff, 1993). Applying this perspective, the prevention of risk involves understanding (1) how the child is functioning in each of the major microsystems of his or her life (e.g., family, school, healthcare system, and neighborhood peer groups), (2) how these major systems interrelate with one another at the mesosystemic level, and (3) how community and societal factors influence the functioning of systems that have a major impact on children (Bronfenbrenner, 1979; Cicchetti & Toth, 1998; Weissberg, Caplan, & Harwood, 1991).

Another key insight derived from prevention research is that health outcomes are determined by the number and severity of risk factors in a person's life, as well as the number and quality of protective factors that mitigate risk (Benson, 1997; Cowen, 1985; Masten & Coatsworth, 1998). Applying this perspective, effective prevention programming involves a balanced approach utilizing strategies that reduce risk and promote competence (Doll & Lyon, 1998; Masten, 2001). For example, several pregnancy prevention programs targeting young adolescent women living in low-income urban and rural neighborhoods have been successful in preventing teenage pregnancy (Frost & Forrest, 1995). Major components of these programs include strategies to reduce risk and to build competencies. Components of these programs that focus primarily on risk reduction include training in (1) abstaining from or delaying sexual activity, (2) successfully using contraceptive devices, and (3) resisting pressure from peers. Components of these programs that focus on the development of competencies include training in (1) problem solving, (2) conflict resolution, and (3) sex education (Jemmott, Jemmott, & Fong, 1998; Vincent, Clearie, & Schluchter, 1987).

Effective prevention programs typically address factors on three levels: (1) the individual child, (2) the contexts in which the child functions, and (3) important relationships in the child's life, including adult relationships with the child and adult-to-adult relationships that can affect children (Durlak, 1997; Pianta & Walsh, 1998). The following is a description of strategies addressing each of these levels of prevention.

Focus on the Individual

Initial efforts in conducting prevention work often focused primarily on increasing children's knowledge, with the assumption that improving knowledge leads to changes in behavior. Unfortunately, programs targeting improvements in knowledge generally have not been effective in achieving successful outcomes (Botvin & Tortu, 1988; Weissberg et al., 1991). In contrast, programs that focus on the development of cognitive, self-regulation, and social skills related to functioning across multiple contexts have been much more effective. Cognitive and academic competence, as well as competence in self-regulation and interpersonal relationships, have been demonstrated repeatedly to be major protective factors in preventing unhealthy patterns of behavior (Masten & Coatsworth, 1998).

Programs designed to improve skills in problem solving, decision making, peer resistance, stress management, and academic performance have been effective in preventing antisocial behavior and health problems (Botvin, Baker, Dusenbury, Tortu, & Botvin, 1990; Elias et al., 1986; Shure & Spivack, 1988; Stephens, 1998). Key components of skills building programs include observing adult and peer models, engaging in role plays, and practicing strategies in real-life contexts (Shure & Spivack, 1988). Incorporating strategies that promote generalization are critical to ensure that the effects of the program produce change across settings and over time (DuPaul & Eckert, 1994).

Focus on the Context

Prevention initiatives have focused substantial effort on improving the quality of parenting. Effective parenting has been shown to involve careful monitoring of children's activities, clear delineation of rules, consistent management of the contingencies for following rules, warmth, and the provision of primarily positive feedback to children (Masten, Best, & Garmezy, 1990; Patterson, Reid, & Dishion, 1992). Successful parenting also includes family involvement in children's education: assisting with homework, providing parent tutoring, encouraging independent reading, and setting high expectations for academic success (Christenson & Sheridan, 2001). Quality of parenting is a protective factor that mitigates biopsychosocial risk and promotes a wide range of healthy outcomes for children (Masten & Coatsworth, 1998).

The school has become a primary target for prevention activities given that children spend such a large proportion of their time in this system, and that schools serve a very high percentage of the general population of children (Dryfoos, 1996). The proliferation of violence in schools and the dramatic rise in the prevalence of sexually transmitted diseases among youth have highlighted the importance of targeting the school as a locus for prevention activities (Centers for Disease Control and Prevention, 1998; Leff et al., 2001). The educational system increasingly has recognized the need to address health issues in school. A primary mission of schools, as delineated by the Goals 2000: Educate America Act (1994), is to remove barriers to instruction by creating safe and drug-free schools.

The nation's schools have engaged in widespread efforts to develop policies and procedures that can prevent the occurrence of violence and drug use in schools. These efforts have included strategies to reduce risk, such as the installation of metal detectors and the education of youth about the adverse consequences of drug use, that have demonstrated limited success (Forgey, Schinke, & Cole, 1997; Hawkins, Farrington, & Catalano, 1998). Comprehensive, asset-building programs that focus on academic and social skills development, careful monitoring of student behavior, and effective teaching and classroom management practices have been shown to be much more effective in promoting safe and healthy behavior among youth (Forgey et al., 1997; Stephens, 1998).

Since the mid-1990s, there has been an increased focus on the quality of children's afterschool activities. During the hours from 3:00 to 7:00 P.M., children, particularly those who are 10 years of age and older, may be left unsupervised by working parents, resulting in increased risk of antisocial behavior, injury, and other health problems (Benson, 1997). Increasingly, prevention efforts have been targeted for youth during these hours of the day. Programs that include academic support and a wide range of recreational activities designed in partnership with youth are being developed to address this need. The dramatic rise in federal funding for these initiatives has contributed greatly to their proliferation across the country, particularly in large urban settings (U.S. Department of Education, 1997).

Focus on Building Relationships

The formation of strong relationships between adults and children, as well as among salient adults from the multiple systems in which children function (e.g., family, school, healthcare system, and community systems), is absolutely essential for positive development. These relationships are illustrated in Figure 7.1.

Developing a caring relationship with a caregiver beginning early in life and continuing throughout childhood and adolescence is perhaps the single most important protective factor in promoting healthy development (Masten, 1994). The attachment between caregiver and child has a major impact not only in addressing children's physical needs but also in developing their cognitive skills and enabling them to learn to regulate emotions and behavior (Carlson & Sroufe, 1995). This attachment also has a strong effect on the child's ability to establish caring, mentoring relationships with adults in multiple contexts, including the school (Pianta, 1997). Disturbances in this relationship, such as the emergence

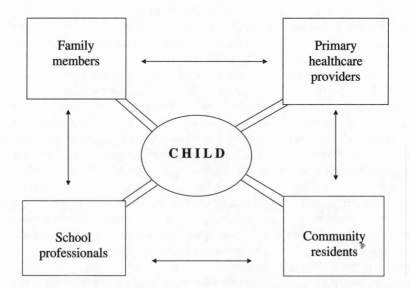

FIGURE 7.1. Important relationships for promoting resilience among children. Parallel lines represent caring, mentoring relationships between adults and the child, and arrows depict partnerships among adults who serve the child.

of a conflictual, mutually coercive relationship in the preschool and elementary school years, is a powerful predictor of antisocial behavior and poor health outcomes in adolescence and adulthood (Patterson et al., 1992).

Although most of the research on adult–child relationships has focused on a caregiver in the home setting, recent research has affirmed the importance of the teacher–student relationship. This relationship can have a significant impact on a child's ability to develop cognitive and academic skills, form successful peer relationships, and learn strategies to regulate emotions and behavior (Pianta, 1999). The importance of the teacher–student relationship is demonstrated in the marked fluctuation of student performance and behavior across grade levels and between classes with different teachers.

Primary healthcare providers serve critical roles in the prevention of health and mental health disorders. The quality of the relationship between primary care provider and patient, including child and family, has been shown to be significantly related to effective outcomes (Kelleher et al., 1997). When a child has a sustained relationship with a pediatric care provider, opportunities for anticipatory guidance arise on a frequent basis. Furthermore, the healthcare provider is in a position to notice initial signs of risk, so that prevention efforts can be targeted to preclude the emergence of serious health and mental health problems.

The prevention of health risk can also be accomplished through the establishment of mentoring relationships with other adults in the community. In schools and in afterschool programs, the involvement of community residents in roles as classroom assistants, tutors, and playground aides can increase the school's (program's) capacity to provide caring, mentoring relationships with students. A particular advantage of these child associates or community partners is that, unlike many of the professional staff, they understand the cultural backgrounds of students, which can facilitate a meaningful relationship with the child and family (Cowen et al., 1996; Dowrick et al., 2001; Fantuzzo, Coolahan, & Weiss, 1997).

The formation of effective working relationships among important adults in the child's life also is critical in the prevention of health risk (Comer, Hayes, Joyner, & Ben-Avie, 1996). The family–school relationship, in particular, has received considerable attention in the research literature. Power and Bartholomew (1987) illustrated how family–school relationships can have a strong impact on the teacher–student relationship. Relationships between parents and teachers that are avoidant and distant may prevent teachers from receiving important information about how to help a child at risk for health problems. Interactions between home and school that are conflictual may reduce the teacher's willingness to form a mentoring relationship with a child who has emerging needs.

The relationship that caregivers develop with primary care health professionals is critical in preventing health risk. Primary care practitioners can serve important roles in educating caregivers for the purpose of preventing health problems, such as obesity, drug and alcohol abuse, sexually transmitted diseases, and injuries (Cheng, DeWitt, Savageau, & O'Connor, 1999). Their effectiveness in this role depends on numerous factors, including the availability of staff to assist with these services and access to third-party reimbursement (Ewing, Selassie, Lopez, & McCutcheon, 1999), but the level of communication between caregiver and healthcare professional is clearly an important consideration.

COMPONENTS OF PROGRAM DEVELOPMENT

Participatory action research methods are highly useful in developing prevention programs that are responsive to the needs of the community. Furthermore, these methods are helpful in linking research with practice (U.S. Department of Health and Human Services, 2001; see Chapter 11). Participatory action research, which is based on methods developed by applied anthropologists, integrates theory based on empirical research with the beliefs and goals of program participants or stakeholders in the development of prevention initiatives (Schensul & Schensul, 1992). A hallmark of this approach is that major stakeholder groups actively collaborate with researchers or prevention specialists in each stage of the process, including program design, implementation, and evaluation (Nastasi et al., 2000). The distinction between participatory action research and applied research or traditional program development and evaluation is described in Table 7.2. The following is a description of some of the major components of the process of program development.

Building Partnerships

At the outset, the prevention specialist needs to identify the major stakeholders of the project and to develop a collaborative relationship with each group (Cowen et al., 1996). Stakeholder groups in schools may include school administrators, general education teachers, special education teachers, related service personnel (e.g., guidance counselors, and nurses), parents, and students. Stakeholders in the community may include mental health providers, primary care providers, faith-based leaders, librarians, staff in afterschool programs, and youth. Stakeholders in a hospital setting may comprise physicians, nursing staff, therapy staff

TABLE 7.2. Distinction between Applied Research and Participatory Action Research

	Applied research	Participatory action research
Authority structure	Hierarchical; researcher has primary authority.	Nonhierarchical; authority shared by project stakeholders.
Goals	Determined by researchers.	Determined by researchers in partnership with stakeholders.
Activities	Designed primarily by research team.	Designed by researchers and stakeholders.
Program integrity	Monitored by research team.	Reviewed in collaboration with program participants.
Outcome measures	Selected by research team.	Adapted in collaboration with program participants.
Data interpretation	Conducted by researchers.	Conducted in partnership with stakeholders.

Note. Applied research refers to program development and evaluation, regardless of whether the project is designed as a formal research initiative.

(e.g., physical therapists, occupational therapists, and speech and language pathologists), social workers, child life staff, patients, and family members.

Prevention specialists based in university settings face unique challenges in developing partnerships with stakeholders in school and community settings. Researchers may differ greatly from school personnel and community residents with regard to their goals and expectations (Fantuzzo & Mohr, 2000). Researchers may view the endeavor as a means to develop a project of national significance, whereas the community may view the program as a service to neighborhood children and families. In addition, researchers implicitly may attempt to control the process of program development and implementation to ensure that the program addresses questions of national significance, and that strategies are implemented with integrity. Operating from a participatory action research framework, it is critical for researchers to establish a nonhierarchical partnership with community-based stakeholders and to support stakeholders in sharing control of the project (Nastasi et al., 2000). This type of arrangement presents some real challenges to researchers, such as an inability to control fully the program agenda and procedures for implementation. The payoff is that, by using these methods, researchers are more likely to develop programs that are acceptable to the community and likely to be sustained. It is noteworthy that even Fast Track, which admittedly used a "top-down" approach in developing program components, incorporated participatory action research methods in adapting prevention procedures in working with specific schools and families (see Conduct Problems Prevention Research Group, 2002).

Creating a Collective Vision

Prevention specialists need to collaborate with major stakeholder groups in developing a collective vision or mission for the project. Creating a shared vision is a dialectical process that considers the needs and intentions of each stakeholder group, including researchers or prevention specialists (Dowrick et al., 2001).

Although the project team may readily agree on the broad focus of the project (e.g., violence prevention, or nutrition education), stakeholders may vary in their views about the program's purpose and intended outcomes. For example, in violence prevention, parents may be interested in reducing violence to protect their children from becoming victims; teachers may have multiple concerns, including the safety of students and of themselves; school administrators may be concerned about the safety of all students and staff members, in addition to the protection of the physical plant; and researchers and policymakers may be interested in studying factors that lead to violence and effective methods of reducing its incidence and impact. Working through disagreements can be useful in sensitizing each stakeholder group about the priorities of other groups. Reaching agreement about the purposes of the project is necessary to delineate a set of common goals and objectives, which in turn can guide the design of project activities and the delineation of outcome indicators.

Co-Constructing the Program

Including major stakeholder groups in the construction of the program from the outset can help to ensure that project methods are perceived by participants as potentially effective, fair, reasonable, and feasible to implement (Nastasi et al., 2000). The full inclusion of multiple stakeholder groups in program planning, however, does not mean that prevention specialists are intended to be passive participants in the co-construction process. Their role is to ensure that the project is designed in a manner consistent with developmental–ecological principles of prevention science, and that research related to the specific focus of prevention efforts is considered. In addition, prevention specialists can serve as advocates for the development of comprehensive programs that include a focus on building the skills of children, changing the contexts in which children operate, and improving important adult-to-child and adult-to-adult relationships in the lives of children. Through ongoing dialogue, the project team can develop a unique prevention initiative that is consistent with theoretical principles and empirically supported strategies described in the research literature, and that is fully endorsed by all the stakeholders who play an active role in the project.

A critical component of program planning is the identification of change agents who can provide services in a competent, developmentally appropriate, and cost-effective manner. Although professional health-care specialists and educators clearly serve important roles in prevention programming, natural helpers have distinct advantages and can serve critical functions to complement these providers. Natural helpers, that is, individuals from the community who are strongly invested in providing support to children, may include parents, grandparents, community residents, older siblings, and peers (Fantuzzo et al., 1997). Natural helpers can readily understand the cultural and linguistic backgrounds of children from their communities, which can be an asset in forming caring, mentoring relationships with them (Cowen et al., 1996). These individuals often are active and successful participants in a network of relationships and are therefore in a position to facilitate the involvement of children and their families into supportive community partnerships. Furthermore, they may be willing to volunteer their time and effort as an investment in the future of their neighborhoods. When professionals collaborate with these community partners, opportunities can be created for the provision of highly effective, culturally competent programs (Dowrick et al., 2001).

Ensuring Program Integrity

A key element of prevention programming is the application of procedures to ensure that the program is implemented as intended. Systematic training at the outset is critical. Because prevention programming may involve professionals and natural helpers in new roles, it is important that training be conducted in a manner that enables these change agents to believe they can be effective in assisting children and their families (Manz, Power, Ginsburg-Block, & Dowrick, 2002). To do so, program providers need to be active participants in the training process by having multiple opportunities to learn and practice skills, and by having an open invitation to question training procedures and to suggest modifications.

The training process must continue throughout the course of programming to respond to unforeseen challenges and to prevent a natural and gradual drift away from standard protocol. There are numerous ways to provide ongoing training. Program providers can meet on a regular basis with the prevention specialist to consider emerging issues and to engage in collaborative problem solving. The project team can co-construct a checklist enumerating the steps that need to be implemented during each session (Ehrhardt, Barnett, Lentz, Stollar, & Reifin, 1996). These checklists can serve as prompts for program providers and also be used to self-monitor intervention integrity. Prevention specialists can observe program sessions or facilitate a process of peer review to offer feedback about program implementation. In addition, sessions can be audio- or videotaped for review at a later time to promote implementation integrity.

Monitoring program integrity can be an anxiety-provoking process that is disempowering to program providers if it is not conducted properly. Developing and refining procedures in partnership with program providers can help in creating a system that effectively maintains integrity, and is useful and acceptable to program providers. For example, explaining the importance of including quality control procedures and dialoguing with providers to identify acceptable strategies for monitoring integrity can be useful.

MODEL PREVENTION INITIATIVES

Many outstanding selective and indicated prevention programs have been developed since the 1950s. The following is a description of some of the programs that exemplify key components of prevention programming.

Primary Mental Health Project: A Model of Community Partnership

The Primary Mental Health Project (PHMP), started in the 1950s by Emory Cowen and colleagues, is an exemplar of a partnership between universities and schools to develop, implement, and evaluate a comprehensive, school-based prevention program (see Cowen et al., 1996). This project has been targeted for elementary-school-age children displaying signs of risk for emotional and behavioral disorders, and therefore is an example of indicated prevention. Children are identified by teacher referral, as well as through a proactive, schoolwide screening process.

A hallmark of this program is the enlistment of natural helpers or child associates as the primary agents of change. Child associates are adults from the community, who typically share the same cultural and linguistic background of the students they serve. Child associates usually volunteer their time to assist at-risk children, although, in some cases, they are paid small stipends. Because of the importance of involving caring, committed, and competent associates, recruitment and selection of these individuals is a high priority for the program. The major goal of PHMP is for child associates to form a meaningful, mentoring relationship with each child assigned to them. Child associates provide support and guidance to children in the context of play activities that are mutually determined by the child and associate. They have also served in roles as facilitators of group programs and therapists for behavior modification programs.

A school-based team consisting of school professionals and child associates meets on a regular basis to develop each child's prevention plan, to monitor progress, and to modify the plan as needed. In this project, the primary role of the mental healthcare professional is to select and train child associates; provide intensive, preservice training to associates; and to offer ongoing consultation to the associates and the school-based prevention team. The ability of this program to be sustained for so many years and be successfully replicated across the country in highly diverse school districts is a testament to the success of the community partnership model and the commitment of project leaders to linking research and practice (see Cowen et al., 1996, for a description of project outcomes).

Pathways: A Model of Participatory Action Research

Pathways, which was initiated in the early 1990s, is a school-based obesity prevention program designed for Native American children attending elementary school (see Davis et al., 1999; Gittelsohn et al., 1999). This population of children was targeted for selective prevention, because it has been shown to be at increased risk for obesity due to a high-fat diet and relatively sedentary lifestyle. This program represents a partnership between universities and schools from several Native American nations. The goal of the collaborative is to design and implement a program that (1) incorporates empirically supported strategies for preventing obesity through diet and physical activity; (2) is responsive to attitudes about diet and exercise among the diverse cultures being served; and (3) is feasible to implement.

A hallmark of this initiative has been the inclusion of important stakeholder groups in defining goals and objectives, and co-constructing the curriculum in partnership with university researchers. These stakeholder groups include students, general education teachers, physical education instructors, school administrators, food service personnel, and parents. A variety of techniques, including focus groups, informal and semistructured interviews, and direct observations of each stakeholder group, have been used to design the program.

The Pathways program has four major components. The nutrition education component, a classroom-based curriculum, incorporates a series of activities, including culturally meaningful stories, adult and peer modeling of nutritious behaviors, role playing, and reinforcement of healthy behavior. Second, in the area of physical activity, children are provided increased opportunities to exercise each week; exercise activities are designed to be responsive to the interests of students; and physical education and recess activities are provided in a systematic, organized manner. Third, training and consultation are provided to food service staff to prepare meals that are highly nutritious, tasty for the children, responsive to the cultural practices of families in the surrounding neighborhoods, and feasible given the constraints of the school systems in which they operate. Fourth, parent training and family support are provided to educate parents about the importance of nutrition and exercise, to provide them with guidelines for preparing healthy meals for children, and to offer strategies for encouraging and reinforcing healthy behaviors at home and in the community. The outcomes of this program are currently under investigation.

Infant Health and Development Program: A Model of Intersystem Collaboration

The Infant Health and Development Program, initiated in the 1980s, is a comprehensive, multisite prevention program targeting low-birth-weight, premature infants and their families (see Infant Health and Human Development Program, 1990). The purpose of this selective prevention program is to prevent health and developmental problems among a population of infants known to be at considerable health risk by virtue of their status at birth.

Infants and families receive a comprehensive program based at home and at a developmental center housing a multidisciplinary staff of educational and health professionals. Shortly after discharge from the hospital following birth and throughout the first year of the child's life, family visits are provided on a weekly basis. The purpose of the visits is to train and empower parents to be effective as the primary educators of their children. Home visitors, who are typically early childhood educators, teach the parents how to promote the development of their child's cognitive, language, and social skills by providing verbal instruction, modeling, and guided practice to parents. In addition, the home visitors offer ongoing social support to families.

In the second and third years of the child's life, programming is provided at a developmental center 5 days per week. The educational staff works with small groups of children on activities to develop cognitive, linguistic, and social skills. Also, in the second and third years of the child's life, parents are provided education at the center regarding child management, social development, and health and safety promotion. Furthermore, opportunities for parents to develop a social support network with other parents and professionals are provided. This program has been demonstrated to be effective in increasing child IQ scores and reducing parent-reported behavior problems by the time children are 3 years of age (Infant Health and Development Program, 1990).

Fast Track: A Model of Comprehensive, Competence-Focused Programming

Developed in the early 1990s, Fast Track is a multisite, school-based program designed to prevent conduct problems among children and adolescents (see Conduct Problems Prevention Research Group, 1999). Based on research that has convincingly demonstrated that multiple biopsychosocial factors contribute to the emergence of antisocial behavior, Fast Track uses a comprehensive, multisystem approach focused on building children's skills and changing the contexts in which they develop. Although Fast Track attempts to reduce the impact of risk, its primary focus is on building protective factors by developing academic and social competencies. Fast Track targets at-risk children upon entry into first grade and maintains programming into adolescence; thus, it is an indicated prevention program, although it also has a universal prevention component (see Chapter 8).

Fast Track has three primary components. The social skills building component is designed to develop friendship-making, conflict resolution, and problem-solving skills. Children are trained through the use of verbal instruction, modeling, role plays, and coaching. With the guidance of trained paraprofessionals, children are provided multiple opportunities to interact with peers in real-life situations to promote the generalization of social skills.

The parent training component is designed to educate parents about methods to manage challenging behaviors, improve the parent–child relationship, and foster collaborative family–school relationships. In addition to group sessions conducted in the school setting, home visits are provided by program staff to promote the generalization of newly acquired parenting skills to the home setting. The academic enrichment component consists of reading tutoring that uses a phonics-based program provided by paraprofessionals twice weekly.

Fast Track also serves as a model for ensuring the integrity of prevention programming. Prevention components are manualized, and staff receive extensive cross-site training before and during the program, and are observed and given feedback on a regular basis. Outcomes after 3 years have demonstrated modest reductions in conduct problems and referrals to special education (Conduct Problems Prevention Research Group, 2002).

CONCLUSIONS

The science and practice of prevention has been strongly influenced by research related to developmental psychopathology and resilience. This research clearly supports a developmental–ecological model of prevention. According to this model, factors contributing to both health risk and resilience emerge in response to a set of complex transactions over extended periods of time between children and the major systems in which they operate. Optimal programming to prevent health risk incorporates strategies that both reduce risk and promote competence.

Applying a developmental–ecological framework, risk reduction and competence promotion strategies need to focus on changing individual children, modifying contexts, and improving relationships. More specifically, prevention strategies should strive to (1) develop children's knowledge and use of cognitive and social skills; (2) change the contexts in which children function, so that they are more conducive to the promotion of cognitive and social skills development; and (3) improve relationships between adults and children, as well as among adults, from the multiple systems in which children function. The formation of strong, caring attachments for children at home and school is very important in preventing health risk. Furthermore, the development of successful partnerships among adults from the family, school, healthcare, and community systems are critical to achieve successful healthcare outcomes.

Principles of participatory action research are highly useful in developing successful prevention programs, and in linking research with practice. In participatory action research, prevention specialists form strong partnerships with community stakeholders and engage them in a collaborative process to balance theory and practice based on empirical research with the values and preferences of each group that has a stake in the program. A hallmark of this approach is that major stakeholders have a critical role in each stage of the project, including the design, implementation, and evaluation stages. By actively involving stakeholders at each stage of the process, the creation of socially valid, culturally meaningful programs is highly likely.

With increased emphasis on prevention since the 1980s, the quality of prevention programming has been accelerating rapidly, although, unfortunately, community-based programming still tends to be more reactive as opposed to proactive and preventive in nature. At this point, state-of-the-art prevention programming involves the following components:

1. Careful consideration of theory based on empirical research, as well as evidence-based prevention strategies.
2. Development of program goals and strategies in partnership with each group that has a stake in the project.
3. A focus on training children in cognitive and social skills, including comprehensive programming for generalization.
4. Inclusion of strategies to improve the ability of the family, school, and healthcare system to promote the development of children.
5. Intensive focus on building caring, mentoring relationships for children in multiple settings.
6. Facilitation of strong, working alliances among adults from the family, school, healthcare, and mental healthcare systems.
7. Incorporation of selective and indicated programs of prevention in the context of an overarching prevention strategy that includes universal programming (see Chapter 8).
8. Comprehensive evaluation of outcomes using formative and summative approaches (see Chapter 9).

There are numerous examples of successful prevention programs at the selective and indicated levels. Most of these initiatives have been funded by foundations and public agencies. For this reason, practitioners seeking to expand the scope of their activities to include prevention work are strongly advised to acquire additional training in grant writing.

REFERENCES

Benson, P. L. (1997). *All kids are our kids: What communities must do to raise caring and responsible children and adolescents*. San Francisco: Jossey-Bass.

Botvin, G. J., Baker, E., Dusenbury, L., Tortu, S., & Botvin, E. M. (1990). Preventing adolescent drug abuse through a multi-modal cognitive-behavioral approach: Results of a 3–year study. *Journal of Consulting and Clinical Psychology, 58,* 437–446.

Botvin, G. J., & Tortu, S. (1988). Preventing adolescent substance abuse through life skills training. In R. H. Price, E. L. Cowen, R. P. Lorion, & J. Ramos-

McKay (Eds.), *14 ounces of prevention: A casebook for practitioners* (pp. 98–110). Washington, DC: American Psychological Association.

Bronfenbrenner, U. (1979). *The ecology of human development.* Cambridge, MA: Harvard University Press.

Caplan, G. (1964). *The principles of preventive psychiatry.* New York: Basic Books.

Carlson, E. A., & Sroufe, L. A. (1995). Contribution of attachment theory to developmental psychology. In D. Cicchetti & D. Cohen (Eds.), *Developmental psychopathology: Vol. 1. Theory and methods* (pp. 581–617). New York: Wiley.

Centers for Disease Control and Prevention. (1998). Trends in sexual risk behaviors among high school students—United States, 1997. *Morbidity and Mortality Weekly Report, 47,* 749–752.

Cheng, T. L., DeWitt, T. G., Savageau, J. A., & O'Connor, K. G. (1999). Determinants of counseling in primary care pediatrics. *Archives of Pediatric and Adolescent Medicine, 53,* 629–633.

Christenson, S. L., & Sheridan, S. M. (2001). *Schools and families: Creating essential connections for learning.* New York: Guilford Press.

Cicchetti, D., & Toth, S. L. (1998). The development of depression in children and adolescents. *American Psychologist, 53,* 221–241.

Comer, J. P., Haynes, N. M., Joyner, E. T., & Ben-Avie, M. (1996). *Rallying the whole village: The Comer process for reforming education.* New York: Teachers College Press.

Conduct Problems Prevention Research Group. (1999). Initial impact of the Fast Track prevention trial for conduct problems: I. The high-risk sample. *Journal of Consulting and Clinical Psychology, 67,* 631–647.

Conduct Problems Prevention Research Group. (2002). The implementation of the Fast Track Program: An example of a large-scale prevention science efficacy trial. *Journal of Abnormal Child Psychology, 30,* 1–18.

Cowen, E. L. (1985). Person centered approaches to primary prevention in mental health: Situation-focused and competence enhancement. *American Journal of Community Psychology, 13,* 31–48.

Cowen, E. L., Hightower, A. D., Pedro-Carroll, J. L., Work, W. C., Wyman, P. A., & Haffey, W. G. (1996). *School-based prevention for children at risk: The primary mental health project.* Washington, DC: American Psychological Association.

Davis, S. M., Going, S. B., Helitzer, D. L., Teufel, N. I., Snyder, P., Gittelsohn, J., Metcalfe, L., Arviso, V., Evans, M., Smyth, M., Brice, R., & Altaha, J. (1999). Pathways: A culturally appropriate obesity-prevention program for American Indian schoolchildren. *American Journal of Clinical Nutrition, 69*(Suppl.), 796S–802S.

Doll, B., & Lyon, M. A. (1998). Risk and resilience: Implications for the delivery of mental health services in the schools. *School Psychology Review, 27,* 348–363.

Dowrick, P. W., Power, T. J., Manz, P. H., Ginsburg-Block, M., Leff, S., Stephen, S., & Kim-Rupnow, S. (2001). Community responsiveness: Examples from under-resourced urban schools. *Journal of Prevention and Intervention in the Community, 21,* 71–90.

Dryfoos, J. G. (1996). *Full-service schools: A revolution in health and social services for children, youth, and families.* San Francisco: Jossey-Bass.

DuPaul, G. J., & Eckert, T. (1994). The effects of social skills curricula: Now you see them, now you don't. *School Psychology Quarterly, 9,* 113–132.

Durlak, J. A. (1997). *Successful prevention programs for children and adolescents.* New York: Plenum Press.

Ehrhardt, K. E., Barnett, D. W., Lentz, F. E., Stollar, S. A., & Reifin, L. H. (1996). Innovative methodology in ecological consultation: Use of scripts to promote treatment acceptability and integrity. *School Psychology Quarterly, 11,* 149–168.

Elias, M. J., Gara, M., Ubriaco, M., Rothbaum, P. A., Clabby, J. F., & Schuyler, T. (1986). Impact of a preventive social problem-solving intervention on children's coping with middle school stressors. *American Journal of Community Psychology, 14,* 259–275.

Ewing, G. B., Selassie, A. W., Lopez, C. H., & McCutcheon, E. P. (1999). Self-report of delivery of clinical preventive services by U.S. physicians: Comparing specialty, gender, age, setting of practice, and area of practice. *American Journal of Preventive Medicine, 17,* 62–72.

Fantuzzo, J. W., Coolahan, K., & Weiss, A. (1997). Resiliency partnership-directed research: Enhancing the social competencies of preschool victims of physical abuse by developing peer resources and community strengths. In D. Cicchetti & S. Toth (Eds.), *Developmental perspective on trauma: Theory, research and intervention* (pp. 463–514). Rochester, NY: University of Rochester Press.

Fantuzzo, J. W., & Mohr, W. (2000). Pursuit of wellness in Head Start: Making beneficial connections for children and families. In D. Cicchetti, J. Rapapport, I. Sandler, & R. Weissberg (Eds.). *The promotion of wellness in children and adolescents* (pp. 341–369). Thousand Oaks, CA: Sage.

Forgey, M. A., Schinke, S., & Cole, K. (1997). *School-based interventions to prevent substance abuse among inner-city minority adolescents.* Washington, DC: American Psychological Association.

Frost, J. J., & Forrest, J. D. (1995). Understanding the impact of effective teenage pregnancy prevention programs. *Family Planning Perspectives, 27,* 188–195.

Gittelsohn, J., Toporoff, E. G., Story, M., Evans, M, Anliker, J., Davis, S., Sharma, A., & White, J. (1999). Food perceptions and dietary behavior of American-Indian children, their caregivers, and educators: Formative assessment findings from Pathways. *Journal of Nutrition Education, 31,* 2–13.

Goals 2000: Educate America Act. (1994). U.S. Congress, Public Law 103–227.

Greenberg, M. T., Domitrovitch, C., & Bumbarger, B. (2001). The prevention of mental disorders in school-aged children: Current state of the field. *Prevention and Treatment, 4*(1), posted March 30, 2001.

Harrell, J. S., Gansky, S. A., McMurray, R. G., Bangdiwala, S. I., Frauman, A. C., & Bradley, C. B. (1998). School-based interventions improve heart health in children with multiple cardiovascular risk factors. *Pediatrics, 102,* 371–380.

Hawkins, J. D., Farrington, D. P., & Catalano, R. F. (1998). Reducing violence through the schools. In D. S. Elliott, B. A. Hamburg, & K. R. Williams (Eds.), *Violence in American schools: A new perspective* (pp. 188–216). Cambridge, UK: Cambridge University Press.

Infant Health and Development Program. (1990). Enhancing the outcomes of low-birth-weight, premature infants: A multi-site, randomized trial. *Journal of the American Medical Association, 263,* 3035–3042.

Institute of Medicine. (1994). *Reducing risks for mental disorders: Frontiers for preventive intervention research.* Washington, DC: National Academy Press.

Jemmott, J. B., Jemmott, L. S., & Fong, G. T. (1998). Abstinence and safer sex: HIV risk-reduction interventions for African American adolescents. *Journal of the American Medical Association, 279,* 1529–1536.

Kelleher, K. J., Childs, G. E., Wasserman, R. C., McInerny, T. K., Nutting, P. A., & Gardner, W. P. (1997). Insurance status and recognition of psychosocial problems: A report from PROS and ASPN. *Archives of Pediatrics and Adolescent Medicine, 151,* 1109–1115.

Leff, S. S., Power, T. J., Manz, P. H., Costigan, T. E., & Nabors, L. A. (2001). School-based aggression prevention programs for young children: Current status and implications for violence prevention. *School Psychology Review, 30,* 344–362.

Loeber, R., & Hay, D. F. (1997). Key issues in the development of aggression and violence from childhood to adulthood. *Annual Review of Psychology, 48,* 371–410.

Manz, P. H., Power, T. J., Ginsburg-Block, M., & Dowrick, P. W. (2002). *Community paraeducators: Improving the effectiveness of urban schools through the engagement and empowerment of low-income, ethnically diverse community residents.* Manuscript submitted for publication.

Masten, A. S. (1994). Resilience in individual development: Successful adaptation despite risk and adversity. In M. Wang & E. Gordon (Eds.), *Risk and resilience in inner city America: Challenges and prospects* (pp. 3–25). Hillsdale, NJ: Erlbaum.

Masten, A. S. (2001). Ordinary magic: Resilience processes in development. *American Psychologist, 56,* 227–238.

Masten, A. S., Best, K. M., & Garmezy, N. (1990). Resilience and development: Contributions for the study of children who overcome adversity. *Development and Psychopathology, 2,* 425–444.

Masten, A. S., & Coatsworth, J. D. (1998). The development of competence in favorable and unfavorable environments: Lessons from research on successful children. *American Psychologist, 53,* 205–220.

Nastasi, B. K., Varjas, K., Schensul, S. L., Silva, K. T., Schensul, J. J., & Ratnayake, P. (2000). The participatory intervention model: A framework for conceptualizing and promoting intervention acceptability. *School Psychology Quarterly, 15,* 207–232.

Natriello, G., McDill, E. L., & Pallas, A. M. (1990). *Schooling disadvantaged children: Racing against catastrophe.* New York: Teachers College Press.

Patterson, G., Reid, J., & Dishion, T. (1992). *Antisocial boys.* Eugene, OR: Castalia.

Pedro-Carroll, J. L., & Cowen, E. L. (1985). The children of divorce intervention program: An investigation of the efficacy of a school-based prevention program. *Journal of Consulting and Clinical Psychology, 53,* 603–611.

Peterson, L., & Oliver, K. K. (1995). Prevention of injuries and disease. In M. C. Roberts (Ed.), *Handbook of pediatric psychology* (2nd ed., pp. 185–199). New York: Guilford Press.

Pianta, R. C. (1997). Adult–child relationship processes and early schooling. *Early Education and Development, 8,* 11–26.

Pianta, R. C. (1999). *Enhancing relationships between children and teachers.* Washington, DC: American Psychological Association.

Pianta, R. C., & Walsh, D. J. (1998). Applying the construct of resilience in schools: Cautions from a developmental systems perspective. *School Psychology Review, 27,* 407–417.

Power, T. J., & Bartholomew, K. L. (1987). Family–school relationship patterns: An ecological assessment. *School Psychology Review, 14,* 222–229.

Ramey, C. T., & Ramey, S. L. (1998). Early intervention and early experience. *American Psychologist, 53,* 109–120.

Sameroff, A. J. (1993). Models of development and developmental risk. In C. H. Zeanah (Ed.), *Handbook of infant mental health* (pp. 3–13). New York: Guilford Press.

Schensul, J. J., & Schensul, S. L. (1992). Collaborative research: Methods of inquiry for social change. In M. D. LeCompte, W. L. Millroy, & J. Preissle (Eds.), *The handbook of qualitative research in education* (pp. 161–200). San Diego: Academic Press.

Shure, M. B., & Spivack, G. (1988). Interpersonal cognitive problem solving. In R. H. Price, E. L. Cowen, R. P. Lorion, & J. Ramos-McKay (Eds.), *14 ounces of prevention: A casebook for practitioners* (pp. 69–82). Washington, DC: American Psychological Association.

Stephens, R. D. (1998). Safe school planning. In D. S. Elliott, B. A. Hamburg, & K. R. Williams (Eds.), *Violence in American schools: A new perspective* (pp. 253–289). Cambridge, UK: Cambridge University Press.

U.S. Department of Education. (1997). *21st Century Community Learning Centers Program.* Washington, DC: Author.

U.S. Department of Health and Human Services. (2001). *Blueprint for change: Research on child and adolescent mental health.* Washington, DC: Department of Health and Human Services, Public Health Service, National Institutes of Health, National Institute of Mental Health.

Vincent, M. L., Clearie, A. F., & Schluchter, M. D. (1987). Reducing adolescent pregnancy through school and community-based education. *Journal of the American Medical Association, 257,* 3382–3386.

Wallerstein, J. S. (1987). Children of divorce: Report of a ten-year follow-up of early latency age children. *American Journal of Orthopsychiatry, 57,* 199–211.

Weissberg, R. P., Caplan, M., & Harwood, R. L. (1991). Promoting competent young people in competence-enhancing environments: A systems-based perspective on primary prevention. *Journal of Consulting and Clinical Psychology, 59,* 830–841.

Williams, C. L., Squillace, M. M., Bollella, M. C., Brotanek, J., Campanaro, L., D'Agostino, C., Pfau, J., Sprance, L., Strobino, B. A., Spark, A., & Boccio, L.

(1998). Healthy Start: A comprehensive health education program for pre-school children. *Preventive Medicine, 27,* 216–223.

Wilson, D. K., Rodrique, J. R., & Taylor, W. C. (Eds.). (1997). *Health-promoting and health-compromising behaviors among minority youth.* Washington, DC: American Psychological Association.

Zigler, E., & Muenchow, S. (1992). *Head Start: The inside story of America's most successful education experiment.* New York: Basic Books.

CHAPTER 8

Developing Universal Prevention Programs

Prevention strategies have been classified into three levels (i.e., indicated, selective, and universal), as described in Chapter 7. Universal prevention involves a systemwide effort to keep individuals healthy and to prevent them from developing unhealthy patterns of behavior. Conceptually, if one successfully applies programs at the universal level, fewer individuals will be in need of programming at the selective or indicated levels. In essence, the strategy is to cast the widest net possible to capture and address the needs of as many individuals as possible, understanding that there will be nonresponders who require other levels of prevention programming (Durlak, 1997).

Because universal prevention programs are designed to address the needs of individuals when they are healthy, and before they display signs of risk, prevention efforts often are targeted on children. In particular, universal prevention programs often focus on key periods of development known to be stressful, such as before or during the transition into elementary school (e.g., Fast Track; see Conduct Problems Prevention Research Group, 2002), or before or during the transition into adolescence (e.g., youth development programs; see Benson, 1997). To capture as many healthy children as possible, universal prevention programs often are provided in schools (Power & Blom-Hoffman, in press), in afterschool programs (Benson, 1997), and in primary care health settings (Kikano, Stange, Flocke, & Zyzanski, 1997).

The hallmark of universal prevention is the building of competence or assets. Efforts are directed at strengthening children's resources, so that they have the resilience to overcome challenges they are likely to encounter during the course of development. In contrast, selective and indicated prevention programs typically are designed to reduce risks and deficits, in addition to promoting competence (see Chapter 7).

171

As with selective and indicated prevention, universal prevention includes a focus on building children's skills, as well as strengthening the systems in which they develop. For universal prevention efforts to be effective, it is not sufficient to impart knowledge and to change belief systems. Participants must have multiple opportunities to practice skills and receive feedback in the actual settings in which they function (Elias et al., 1997). For this reason, it is important that prevention programming be infused in all aspects of the child's life, including classroom learning environment, lunchroom and playground context, afterschool program, and family.

Critical domains of skills building are the areas of cognitive/academic functioning and social/emotional functioning (Masten & Coatsworth, 1998). A major focus of efforts to promote academic success has been to promote literacy skills acquisition in the preschool and early elementary school years (see Torgesen, 2002), although the development of academic skills clearly is essential throughout elementary, middle, and secondary school. Efforts to promote social and emotional development have focused on providing instruction, modeling, and opportunities for guided practice to children in the areas of empathy, problem solving, communication, and emotion regulation (see Conduct Problems Prevention Research Group, 2002; Payton et al., 2000).

Universal prevention efforts also have been directed at increasing knowledge, changing beliefs, and improving skills related to specific domains of health behavior. For example, prevention programs designed to improve health behaviors related to sexual activity and to reduce the risk of HIV have focused on increasing children's knowledge about HIV, changing beliefs about the acceptability of prevention methods (e.g., abstinence and condom use), and enhancing skills in using prevention procedures (see Jemmott, Jemmott, & Fong, 1998). Likewise, programs designed to improve cardiovascular health have incorporated classroom-based instructional programs to educate children about selecting healthy foods, engaging in physical exercise on a regular basis, and coping with the pressure to smoke cigarettes (see Harrell et al., 1998).

Because cognitive and social/emotional development occurs in the context of systems that have a powerful influence on behavior (Sameroff, 1993), successful universal prevention programs examine systems issues and facilitate the healthy development of children in one or more contexts. In this chapter, we describe factors related to the family, school, community, and healthcare systems that can promote the healthy development of children and, therefore, ought to be considered in designing universal prevention programs. Next, we describe examples of effective or promising universal prevention programs that utilize a competence-promoting approach at both the child and systems levels.

SYSTEMIC FACTORS THAT PROMOTE COMPETENCE

The following section describes factors within the family, school, community, and healthcare systems that can have a strong influence on the development of healthy patterns of behavior. These factors, which are summarized in Table 8.1, are important to consider in designing universal prevention programs for children. Our position is that comprehensive, potentially effective universal prevention programs include factors related to these systems of development.

Family Factors

To state the obvious, well-functioning families within which there are strong parent–child relationships are contexts that promote the development of healthy children. Research related to resilience has indicated clearly that a strong attachment to a primary caregiver is essential to promoting healthy development (Masten & Coatsworth, 1998). A sustained, caring, secure relationship with a caregiver has been shown to influence the developing child's motivation to achieve academically and ability to regulate emotions, which is critical for successful social relationships (Cicchetti, Toth, & Lynch, 1995; Greenberg, Speltz, & DeKlyen, 1993). The development of strong caregiver–child relationships has been shown to have an effect on the quality of relationships with teachers and other adults in the community, as well as with peers (Pianta, 1999). Fail-

TABLE 8.1. Systemic Factors That Promote the Healthy Development of Children

Family factors	Caregiver–child attachment
	Effective parenting skills
	Supportive social network
	Emotionally healthy caregivers
School factors	Teacher–child relationships
	Quality of instruction
	Professional support for teachers
	Collaborative family–school relationships
Community factors	Mentoring relationships with community members
	Availability of enjoyable, enriching programs
	Coordination of community agencies
Health system factors	Sustained relationship with a health provider
	Accessibility of services
	Collaboration between healthcare and school systems

ure to develop secure attachments, or a major disruption in these relationships, is a risk factor for compromised developmental outcomes, including school failure, aggression and/or victimization by peers, and psychopathology.

Effective parenting skills can promote warm, enriching parent–child relationships and enable families to manage conflicts with respect and creativity. For example, the use of behavior management strategies that emphasize positive reinforcement for adaptive behavior as opposed to punishment for nonadaptive behavior can be highly successful and promote positive family relationships. Being strategic in the use of positive reinforcement, including caregiver attention and praise, by providing positive reinforcement contingent upon responsible behavior, and withholding reinforcement in response to irresponsible behavior, is highly effective in shaping children's behavior. Also, parenting that involves delivering corrective feedback to children in a calm manner, with brief directives about how to behave in the future, is more effective than giving emotionally laden reprimands that focus on children's deficits (see Hembree-Kigin & McNeil, 1995).

Caregivers involved in social networks with other caregivers to provide emotional support and share knowledge about child development generally are more effective in parenting their children than those who are socially isolated (Wahler & Dumas, 1989). Caregivers engaged in mutually supportive relationships with their spouses or partners typically are more effective parents than those who engage in conflictual dyadic relationships. Furthermore, caregivers who are able to function competently as adults in home, community, and occupational settings are likely to be successful in developing and maintaining caring and secure attachments with their children (Campbell, 1994).

School Factors

Schools have enormous potential to promote healthy patterns of behavior and to protect children from health risks (Doll & Lyon, 1998; Power & Blom-Hoffman, in press). Schools are a workshop for children to develop their cognitive abilities and academic skills. Through successful performance in school, children learn to view themselves as competent individuals who have control over the outcomes of their performance. Furthermore, schools provide children numerous opportunities on a daily basis to learn effective ways to form relationships with other children and to resolve conflicts when they arise (Lewis, Sugai, & Colvin, 1998).

Successful performance in school, both academically and socially, is related, in part, to the relationships children have with their teachers (Pianta, 1999). When children are engaged in warm and caring relationships with teachers, and when teachers and children can address academic and behavioral difficulties in a way that does not undermine their relationship, children are more likely to achieve academic success and to relate to their peers effectively.

The quality of children's instruction in school is obviously critical to academic success. Children typically learn more rapidly when materials are at the proper instructional level, ensuring that the proportion of familiar to unfamiliar information during instruction is at an appropriate level (Shapiro, 1996). Learning also depends upon the amount of classroom time devoted to instruction and the level of student engagement in learning activities (Gettinger & Seibert, 2002).

Quality of teaching is related to many variables, but a critical factor is the support provided to teachers in coping with challenges related to their professional activities. Providing teachers opportunities for professional development and career enhancement can help to sustain their motivation and commitment. Creating a context in which teachers are supported by the administrative staff and involved in a supportive network with colleagues can assist them in coping with professional demands (Maslach & Leiter, 1997). Furthermore, providing health promotion activities for educational staff in schools can help them to develop healthy lifestyles, cope with stress more effectively, and model for students healthy patterns of behavior (Talley & Short, 1995).

Effective schools are responsive to the values and needs of families residing in the surrounding neighborhoods (Comer, Haynes, Joyner, & Ben-Avie, 1996). The diverse cultural and linguistic backgrounds of families living in the community are well represented among the staff working in the school. In successful schools, the educational staff, regardless of their cultural backgrounds, interact effectively with children and families from the diverse backgrounds reflected in the community. Furthermore, the schools are closely connected with formal and informal agencies in the community involved in the education of children through afterschool programs (Benson, 1997).

Family involvement in education repeatedly has been shown to have an effect on children's success in school (Christenson & Sheridan, 2001). Family involvement includes activities in which families engage within and outside the home to support the education of their children, including homework assistance, parent tutoring, and trips to parks and museums. Family involvement also refers to caregiver participation in school-based activities (e.g., participating in parent–teacher organizations, and volunteering to assist with field trips and career days). In addition, family involvement includes the quality of communications between the family and school, and the extent to which parents and teachers are able to collaborate to resolve challenges that children experience in their development (Epstein, 1995; Fantuzzo, Tighe, & Childs, 2000).

Community Factors

Agencies in the community provide many programs that support the healthy development of children. In fact, some families prefer to seek out services from informal agencies in the community than through formal institutions, such as hospitals, clinics, or schools (Tucker, 2002). These informal agencies include youth sports leagues, faith-based organizations, libraries, afterschool programs, food cooperatives, and public housing projects (Freudenberg, 2000). Examples of the domains of health promotion addressed through informal agencies are presented in Table 8.2.

Community-based agencies help to orchestrate neighborhood resources to address important developmental needs of children. These agencies may provide children with opportunities to engage in diverse recreational activities with peers of similar age, such as through sports leagues, dance troupes, and book clubs. They often afford children opportunities to become engaged in meaningful, supervised activities during afterschool hours, when primary caregivers are less available and the risk of antisocial and unhealthy patterns of behavior is heightened (U.S. Department of Education, 1997).

Neighborhood organizations provide a context within which children can form mentoring relationships with adults and older peers. In situations in which children are not able to form meaningful attachments with a primary caregiver in the family, the mentoring relationships they form through community agencies may be vital in protecting them from developmental risks. Alternatively, for children who have been successful in forming strong family-based attachments, mentors in the community may increase their resilience and enable them to cope successfully during adolescent transition points, when it is important to individuate from primary caregivers and make decisions outside the family (see Benson, 1997).

Although the informality of community organizations can be an asset with regard to engaging youth and promoting caring relationships, the lack of structure may limit the degree of coordination among agencies. Creating networks of informal community organizations and linking them with formal institutions can help to ensure that children's needs are being addressed and that services are being coordinated (Stone, 1996). For example, initiatives designed to coordinate educational ef-

TABLE 8.2. Examples of the Health Promotion Domains
Addressed through Informal Community Agencies

Youth sport leagues	Fitness education
	Nutrition education
	Social skills development
	Drug and alcohol prevention
	Violence prevention
	Injury prevention
Faith-based organizations	Literacy programming
	Academic tutoring
	Social skills development
	Responsible sexual behavior
	Drug and alcohol prevention
	Violence prevention
Library	Literacy programming
	Academic tutoring
	Nutrition education
	Drug and alcohol prevention
	Violence prevention
	Injury prevention
Afterschool programs	Literacy programming
	Academic tutoring
	Social skills development
	Drug and alcohol prevention
	Violence prevention
Food cooperatives	Nutrition education
	Fitness education
	Drug and alcohol prevention
Public housing projects	Parent education
	Nutrition education
	Fitness education
	Responsible sexual behavior
	Drug and alcohol prevention
	Violence prevention

forts in school, in afterschool programs, and at home may strengthen the
community's capacity to education its children and lead to better educational outcomes (Comer et al., 1996).

Health System Factors

Primary healthcare is an important venue for the promotion of children's
health. Primary care provides a mechanism for treating illnesses when
they arise and has the potential for preventing the occurrence of disease

(Cohen, Halvorson, & Gosselink, 1994). Although there are numerous barriers to the provision of preventive services in primary care settings (e.g., lack of time, lack of reimbursement for prevention activities, insufficient education of providers), several groups have been successful in addressing these problems and providing effective prevention services (e.g., Goodson, Gotlieb, & Smith, 1999).

Ensuring that children have access to a primary healthcare provider is clearly an important health promotion strategy. Furthermore, promoting the formation of continuous, caring relationships between primary healthcare providers and children, as well as their families, is important in fostering healthy development and preventing disease (Kelleher et al., 1997). Through sustained relationships, primary care providers are in an advantageous position to advocate for their patients, anticipate potential problems and recommend prevention practices, and engage in partnerships to manage illnesses collaboratively when they arise (see Chapter 5).

Although the healthcare system often works in isolation from the school and community agencies, more successful healthcare can often be provided when the healthcare system is connected with these other systems. For example, facilitating collaboration between primary healthcare providers and school professionals in developing an individualized asthma management program is an effective and feasible approach to managing pediatric asthma (Lwebuga-Mukasa & Dunn-Georgiou, 2002). Likewise, collaborations between healthcare and school professionals can be highly effective in designing comprehensive health promotion programs (see Davis et al., 1999).

MODEL UNIVERSAL PREVENTION PROGRAMS

Many exemplary universal prevention programs have been developed and evaluated over the years. These programs span several broad domains, including the prevention of sexually transmitted diseases (STDs), the promotion of cardiovascular health, the development of early literacy skills, and the prevention of aggressive and violent behavior. The following is a description of evidence-based, universal prevention programs that address these domains. We also include a brief description of an initiative designed to promote the selection and use of effective and useful strategies for promoting children's health and social development.

Be Proud! Be Responsible!: Preventing Sexually Transmitted Diseases

Be Proud! Be Responsible! is a universal prevention program that has primarily targeted African American youth attending middle schools in inner-city settings for the purpose of promoting responsible sexual behavior and preventing the risk of STD, including HIV infection (see Jemmott, Jemmott, & Fong, 1992).

A hallmark of the program is that the content and process of the training experiences are highly responsive to the cultural values of the community and the interests of participating youth. Groups are facilitated by African American adults or older peers attending local high schools. The program typically is offered on two consecutive Saturdays over an 8-hour period. Sessions are designed to be educational, entertaining, and culturally sensitive, incorporating the use of videos, games, group discussions, and experiential exercises. The training modules emphasizes the theme of being proud and responsible by encouraging youth to (1) be proud of themselves and their community, (2) behave in a responsible manner for their own good and for the sake of the community, (3) consider the goals they have for their lives, and (4) reflect on how unhealthy patterns of behavior can thwart the achievement of goals. The intervention incorporates educational and cognitive-behavioral strategies to promote changes in attitude and behavior (for a further description of program procedures, see Jemmott et al., 1992).

The Be Proud! Be Responsible! program has been developed and evaluated for use with an abstinence as well as a safer sex approach to responsible sexual behavior (see Jemmott et al., 1998). The abstinence approach emphasizes abstinence from sex as a way to prevent the risk of pregnancy and STD, including HIV. A major focus of the abstinence curriculum is to increase skills and self-efficacy regarding one's ability to negotiate abstinence and to resist peer pressure. The safer sex approach affirms that abstinence is the safest approach, but that using condoms can be effective in reducing the risk of pregnancy and STD if students were to engage in sex. The emphasis of the safer sex curriculum is to increase skills and self-efficacy in the use of condoms and to allay fears that condom use reduces sexual enjoyment.

Randomized clinical research trials have been conducted to evaluate the efficacy of the abstinence versus the safer sex approach in relation to a control group provided with a generic health promotion program delivered in a culturally sensitive manner (Jemmott et al., 1998). Outcome data related to youth self-reports of sexual intercourse, condom use, and unprotected sexual intercourse were collected at 3 months, 6 months, and 12 months following intervention. The results demonstrated that both approaches can reduce the risk of behaviors associated with risk for STD; however, the safer sex approach generally had more lasting effects. The safer sex approach was more effective than the abstinence method in reducing unprotected sexual intercourse, suggesting that the safer sex approach may be more effective among youth who are sexually experienced. The data failed to indicate that educating youth about condom use increases sexual activity. It is noteworthy that the adult and peers trainers were equally effective with regard to achieving intervention effects.

Child and Adolescent Trial for Cardiovascular Health (CATCH): Promoting Cardiovascular Health

CATCH, a comprehensive, schoolwide prevention program for elementary-school-age children, is designed to prevent cardiovascular disease (see Leupker et al., 1996). CATCH has three basic components: (1) modification of the meals served to children in school; (2) enhanced activity in physical education classes; and (3) classroom-based instruction regarding diet, exercise, and the harmful effects of cigarette smoking (for older elementary school students). The food service intervention, known as Eat Smart, involves serving tasty meals at recommended levels of nutrition, while substantially reducing the intake of fat, saturated fat, and sodium. The exercise component consists of introducing a moderate-to-vigorous level of exercise in physical education classes. The classroom curriculum provides education and opportunities for skills building related to healthy patterns of eating and exercise.

This program also includes a family education component. Caregivers are provided with activity packets that complement the school curriculum and encourage the family to implement core elements of the program in the home. Each year of the program, about six packets are sent home for families to work on together. Also, children and families are invited to participate in a fun night, involving a dance performance by students, stations providing nutritious snacks, and booths through which recipes for tasty and nutritious meals are distributed.

The outcomes of CATCH have been evaluated through a large, multisite clinical trial involving 96 schools (Luepker et al., 1996). Schools were randomly assigned to one of three groups: CATCH including the family component of the program, CATCH not including the family component, and a control group receiving the standard food service, physical education, and health education programs provided through the school. Children were enrolled in the study in third grade and maintained in the project through fifth grade. Outcomes were evaluated at two levels. The school-level assessment consisted of evaluations of the fat content of lunches served in the school and the amount of moderate-to-vigorous activity demonstrated in physical education classes. The individual student assessment involved monitoring serum cholesterol and blood pressure levels, measuring body mass, and examining self-reports of eating and exercise patterns.

The findings demonstrated that the percentage of intake from fat was lower and the amount of moderate-to-vigorous exercise was higher among children in CATCH compared to the control group. Also, self-reports of daily intake of fat were lower, and self-reports of moderate-to-vigorous exercise were higher among children in CATCH than for those in the control group. However, blood pressure, body mass, and cholesterol levels did not differ between the treatment and control groups. Furthermore, the family education component of CATCH generally did not add to the effect of CATCH, suggesting that this component may need to be provided in a more intensive and systematic manner to contribute to intervention effects.

This study demonstrates that it is possible to change the diet and exercise patterns of children through a school-based prevention program, in a manner that does not require a substantial investment of fiscal and personnel resources. However, the study raises questions about the ability of the program to change biological markers of physical health. More intensive programming with the family and the involvement of communitywide efforts of prevention, including interventions using the mass media and efforts targeting grocery stores and youth programs, may be needed to achieve effects in biological indicators of health status. Also, the evaluation of follow-up effects 3 to 5 years after intervention may be necessary to demonstrate change at the biological level.

Success for All: Promoting Literacy Development

The development of reading skills has been identified as a major public health issue by the National Institute of Child Health and Human Development (NICHD: Lyon, 2002). Children who cannot read at an acceptable level are at increased risk for school dropout, unhealthy patterns of behavior, and failure to perform competently in the occupational arena as adults (Lyon, Alexander, & Yaffe, 1997). Because the trajectory of reading failure typically is established in the early elementary school years (Juel, 1988), and because it is estimated that 37% of children are inadequate readers by fourth grade (National Center for Educational Statistics, 2001), targeting literacy initiatives for children in kindergarten through third grade has become a national priority.

A voluminous body of accumulated research identifies key elements of reading instruction in the early elementary school years (see Torgesen, 2002, for a useful review of this literature). At this point, it is very clear that a balanced, multicomponent approach to literacy development is the most effective way to teach reading to all children. The National Reading Panel (2000) of NICHD indicated that the components of effective reading instruction for all children include an emphasis on (1) phonemic awareness and decoding skills, (2) fluency in word recognition and text processing skills, (3) reading comprehension, (4) oral language vocabulary, (5) spelling, and (6) writing.

Numerous literacy programs that use a balanced, multicomponent approach have been developed and validated for use with young elementary-school-age children. One of the most widely used programs, Success for All (Slavin & Madden, 2001), has been developed primarily for children from low-income neighborhoods in urban and rural settings. Success for All has four major components, reflecting a balanced approach to reading instruction: (1) teaching reading in the context of having children read meaningful text, (2) providing explicit instruction in phonemic awareness and decoding, (3) focusing on reading comprehension, and (4) teaching metacognitive strategies, including error detection and correction strategies. (See Slavin and Madden, 2001, for a detailed description of the goals and procedures of this program.)

Although Success for All has been designed for use in general education settings with all children, this program includes an intensive tutorial component for students who are struggling with reading and need additional assistance. An advantage of the tutoring component is that it is closely integrated with the general education program.

The outcomes of this program have been studied extensively in schools from various regions of the country (see Slavin & Madden, 2001). The studies generally use a quasi-experimental design, with the outcomes for targeted schools being compared with those from comparison schools with similar demographic characteristics. Outcome measures include standardized, norm-referenced tests of various components of reading skill, although some studies have used state- or district-administered tests (Hurley, Chamberlain, Slavin, & Madden, 2000). In general, students enrolled in schools that use Success for All have been shown to read 2.5 months higher in grade equivalents than those from control schools by the end of first grade. By the end of fifth grade, the difference between targeted and control children has been demonstrated to be 1.1 years in grade equivalents (Slavin & Madden, 2001). Furthermore, several studies have shown that Success for All can successfully reduce placement in special education (Smith, Ross, & Casey, 1994).

Success for All is intended to be used in combination with other components as part of a comprehensive, schoolwide reform program, referred to as Roots and Wings (Slavin, Madden, & Wasik, 1997). These additional program components include evidence-based practices in math, writing, science, and social studies; progress monitoring of academic skills development; effective strategies of classroom management; professional development of educational staff; family support and parental involvement in education; and school management involving the development, implementation, and evaluation of a schoolwide reform plan.

Second Step: Promoting Social Competence and Preventing Aggression

Second Step is a widely used prevention program designed to increase competence in core areas of social and emotional development for the purpose of systematically reducing aggressive behavior, which has been demonstrated to be predictive of antisocial behavior in adolescence and adulthood (Cairns, Cairns, Neckerman, Ferguson, & Gariepy, 1989). Second Step is principally designed for implementation in school settings, although it can be adapted for use in afterschool programs. This program is intended for children in prekindergarten through middle school (Committee for Children, 1991, 1992, 1997).

Second Step targets domains of competence that are critical to effective emotional and social development, including empathy, social problem solving, and anger management (see Frey, Hirschstein, & Guzzo, 2000, for a detailed description of this prevention initiative). Empathy refers to the ability to identify, understand, and respond to the emotions of others. Social problem solving is a five-step process involving skills in (1) identifying the problem, (2) brainstorming solutions, (3) evaluating potential solutions, (4) selecting and implementing a plan, and (5) evaluating the chosen solution. Anger management entails identifying triggers that arouse anger and developing self-talk strategies to reduce emotionality and reflect on the situation.

Second Step typically is taught to children in the classroom twice weekly during the course of the year. The program is intended for continuous use throughout the preschool, elementary, and middle school years. Teachers are trained to use a variety of instructional strategies, including didactic presentation with visual aides, video-based lessons, student discussions, modeling, role plays, and opportunities to solve real issues that arise in school.

Second Step places a strong emphasis on creating a school and classroom environment that promotes social and emotional development. Program trainers collaborate with building principals to identify strategies to create a school atmosphere to promote the learning of core competencies. Principals are encouraged to advocate for the program during faculty meetings, model program competencies in their interactions with faculty and students, and hold teachers accountable for following program lesson plans. Teachers are guided to create a classroom climate that supports the achievement of program goals by modeling core competencies throughout the day and reinforcing students for spontaneously applying the skills targeted by this program (Frey et al., 2000).

Second Step also includes a component for families to elicit the support of caregivers in the program and to promote the generalization of social skills to out-of-school settings. The program for families includes six video-based modules to assist with program instruction.

The effectiveness of this program for students in second and third grade has been evaluated in a well-designed study with an experimental design (Grossman et al., 1997). Twelve participating schools were paired on the basis of important demographic characteristics. One school from each pair was randomly assigned to Second Step, and the other school in the pair to a control group that received instruction in skills not directly targeted by Second Step (e.g., self-esteem). Children were instructed twice weekly over the course of a 4- to 5-month period. Outcome measures included direct observations of behavior in the classroom, lunchroom, and playground settings, as well as teacher and parent reports of behavior.

The findings revealed that children in Second Step demonstrated significantly fewer observed acts of physical aggression than those in the control group. A similar, although nonsignificant, trend was demonstrated for observations of verbal hostility. The differences between groups were most noticeable in the lunchroom and playground settings as opposed to the classroom context. The clinical significance of the findings is quite compelling: Children in Second Step demonstrated 1.1 fewer acts of physical aggression and 17.1 more acts of neutral or prosocial behavior per hour per student in the lunchroom and playground settings than those in the control group. Furthermore, the effects generally were maintained for 6 months following treatment. However, parent and teacher ratings of behavior did not demonstrate significant differences between groups. The researchers speculated that parents and teachers may not be aware of the subtle changes taking place in student behavior in response to Second Step, particularly in the lunchroom/playground contexts. However, they admitted that the failure of adults to report changes in response to the program may have an effect on the acceptability of Second Step, which could reduce their willingness and motivation to sustain involvement in the program. Strategies to improve the social validity of Second Step for teachers and parents may need to be developed further in the future.

Collaborative to Advance Social and Emotional Learning (CASEL): Promoting and Disseminating Effective Prevention Programs

CASEL is an international advocacy organization that promotes social and emotional learning as an essential approach to maintain and improve the health status of children in preschool through high school (Payton et al., 2000). CASEL strives to coordinate the efforts of schools and other community agencies to identify and implement integrated programs of health promotion. Given that the risk and protective factors of many health problems (e.g., substance abuse, violence, STD, psychopathology) are very similar, CASEL provides a framework for designing a comprehensive prevention program to address the healthcare needs of children and their families. The major goals of CASEL are to (1) promote scientific inquiry into social and emotional learning; (2) facilitate the translation of research into practice, particularly in educational settings; (3) disseminate information about research-based strategies to promote social and emotional learning; (4) improve the training of education professionals related to their ability to provide programs to promote social and emotional learning; and (5) establish partnerships among researchers, clinicians, educators, community members, and policymakers (Payton et al., 2000).

One of the primary contributions of CASEL has been the delineation of a set of core competencies that characterize effective health promotion programs (see Elias et al., 1997). The identification of these competencies was based on a comprehensive review of theories of social development and behavior change, as well as the empirical literature related to child and systems factors that promote healthy outcomes for children. The key competencies of social and emotional learning are clustered into four broad areas: (1) awareness of self and others, including the ability to monitor and regulate feelings and the ability to take the perspective of others; (2) respect for self and others, involving the intention to lead a healthy lifestyle and a commitment to value others and to treat them fairly; (3) responsible decision making, including the capacity to set reasonable goals for behavior and to develop, implement, and evaluate a plan to achieve these goals; and (4) social interaction skills, referring to the ability to cooperate with others, resolve conflicts, and resist peer pressure.

The CASEL team has developed checklists based on these competencies to assist professionals in evaluating the extent to which prevention programs address critical issues that have been demonstrated to promote social and emotional learning (Payton et al., 2000). Using these rating scales, consultants can evaluate when the program meets each core competency on a scale from 0 (does not address the competency) to 3 (provides opportunities for children to learn the competency and to apply it in actual settings).

Another important contribution of CASEL has been the delineation of critical elements of effective prevention programs. These elements, which are described briefly in Table 8.3, include aspects of program design, program coordination, educator preparation and support, and program evaluation. With regard to program design, it is important that programs be grounded in well-developed theory and empirical research. The curriculum should be linked closely with goals and objectives based on the conceptual model and prepared in a sequential manner, with clearly specified learning activities. Also, it is critical that prevention training be infused into the educational curriculum across subject areas and school settings (e.g., classroom, playground, lunchroom). Program coordination involves the development of a school context that supports the prevention initiative and the creation of partnerships with the community and with families to promote children's health. Professional support is an essential aspect of effective prevention programs; the educational staff need to be appropriately trained and provided with ongoing support to be successful in delivery the health promotion program. Finally, schools and community agencies should select programs that have been validated by well-designed empirical studies. CASEL has developed techniques that are useful in evaluating the extent to which prevention programs incorporate these components of effective programming.

The CASEL team is strongly committed to the dissemination of information that can be useful in developing, selecting, implementing, and evaluating programs that can be effective in promoting social and emotional learning. One of their main vehicles to do this is through their website at *www.casel.org*.

TABLE 8.3. Elements of Effective Prevention Programs Outlined by CASEL

Program design	Well-developed conceptual model Sequential curriculum Clarity of session objectives and learning activities Infusion of curriculum across subject areas Useful techniques to ensure quality control
Program coordination	Creation of school climate that supports classroom learning Strengthening of family–school partnerships Strengthening of school–community linkages
Professional support	Systematic training of educators Ongoing support and technical assistance to educators
Program evaluation	Well-designed study to evaluate effectiveness Empirical data to support effectiveness of program

Note. For a more detailed description, see Payton et al. (2000).

CONCLUSIONS

Universal prevention, because it targets healthy children for the purpose of maintaining and enhancing their development and welfare, is a competence-promoting enterprise. Effective prevention programs attempt to promote change at two levels. At the level of the individual, they are designed to improve knowledge, change attitudes, and facilitate skills acquisition in real-life settings. At the level of systems, successful programs create contexts that promote cognitive development, and social and emotional learning. These programs strengthen children's attachments in families, in communities, in schools, and in healthcare, and they facilitate collaborative linkages among these systems.

Model universal prevention programs have been established to address a broad range of health concerns, including pregnancy and STD, the use of alcohol and drugs, cardiovascular disease, and antisocial behavior. A thorough examination of the risk and protective factors of these health issues has revealed a common set of factors that promote children's health and prevent the risk of disease. For this reason, prevention efforts in schools and communities should be carefully coordinated, so that they complement each other and use resources in an efficient manner.

REFERENCES

Benson, P. L. (1997). *All kids are our kids: What communities must do to raise caring and responsible children and adolescents.* San Francisco: Jossey-Bass.

Cairns, R. B., Cairns, B. D., Neckerman, H. J., Ferguson, L. L., & Gariepy, J. L. (1989). Growth and aggression: I. Childhood to early adolescence. *Developmental Psychology, 25,* 320–330.

Campbell, S. B. (1994). Hard-to-manage preschool boys: Externalizing behavior, social competence, and family context at two-year follow-up. *Journal of Abnormal Child Psychology, 22,* 147–166.

Christenson, S. L., & Sheridan, S. M. (2001). *Schools and families: Creating essential connections for learning.* New York: Guilford Press.

Cicchetti, D., Toth, S. L., & Lynch, M. (1995). Bowlby's dream comes full circle: The application of attachment theory to risk and psychopathology. In T. H. Ollendick & R. J. Prinz (Eds.), *Advances in clinical child psychology* (Vol. 17; pp. 1–75). New York: Plenum Press.

Cohen, S. J., Halvorson, H. W., & Gosselink, C. A. (1994). Changing physician behavior to improve disease prevention. *Preventive Medicine, 23,* 284–291.

Comer, J. P., Haynes, N. M., Joyner, E. T., & Ben-Avie, M. (1996). *Rallying the whole village: The Comer process for reforming education.* New York: Teachers College Press.

Committee for Children. (1991). *Second Step: A violence prevention curriculum; Preschool—kindergarten*. Seattle: Author.

Committee for Children. (1992). *Second Step: A violence prevention curriculum; Grades 1–3*. Seattle: Author.

Committee for Children. (1997). *Second Step: A violence prevention curriculum; Middle school/junior high*. Seattle: Author.

Conduct Problems Prevention Research Group. (2002). The implementation of the Fast Track program: An example of a large-scale prevention science efficacy trial. *Journal of Abnormal Child Psychology, 30,* 1–18.

Davis, S. M., Going, S. B., Helitzer, D. L., Teufel, N. I., Snyder, P., Gittelsohn, J., Metcalfe, L., Arviso, V., Evans, M., Smyth, M., Brice, R., & Altaha, J. (1999). Pathways: A culturally appropriate obesity-prevention program for American Indian schoolchildren. *American Journal of Clinical Nutrition, 69*(Suppl.), 796S–802S.

Doll, B., & Lyon, M. A. (1998). Risk and resilience: Implications for the delivery of mental health services in the schools. *School Psychology Review, 27,* 348–363.

Durlak, J. A. (1997). *Successful prevention programs for children and adolescents.* New York: Plenum Press.

Elias, M. J., Zins, J., Weissberg, R. P., Frey, K., Greenberg, M. T., Haynes, N., Kessler, R., Schwab-Stone, M., & Shriver, T. P. (1997). *Promoting social and emotional learning: Guidelines for educators.* Alexandria, VA: Association for Supervision and Curriculum Development.

Epstein, J. L. (1995). School/family/community partnerships: Caring for the children we share. *Phi Delta Kappan, 76,* 701–712.

Fantuzzo, J., Tighe, E., & Childs, S. (2000). Family Involvement Questionnaire: A multivariate assessment of family participation in early childhood education. *Journal of Educational Psychology, 92,* 367–376.

Freudenberg, N. (2000). Health promotion in the city: A review of current practice and future prospects in the United States. *Annual Review of Public Health, 21,* 473–503.

Frey, K. S., Hirschstein, M. K., & Guzzo, B. A. (2000). Second Step: Preventing aggression by promoting social competence. *Journal of Emotional and Behavioral Disorders, 8,* 102–112.

Gettinger, M., & Seibert, J. K. (2000). Best practices in increasing academic learning time. In A. Thomas & J. Grimes (Eds.), *Best practices in school psychology IV.* Bethesda, MD: National Association of School Psychologists.

Goodson, P., Gotleib, N. H., & Smith, M. M. (1999). Put prevention into practice: Evaluation of program initiation of nine clinical sites. *Journal of Preventive Medicine, 17,* 73–78.

Greenberg, M. T., Speltz, M. L., & DeKlyen, M. (1993). The role of attachment in the early development of disruptive behavior disorders. *Development and Psychopathology, 5,* 191–213.

Grossman, D. C., Neckerman, H. J., Koepsell, T. D., Liu, P. Y., Asher, K. N., Beland, K., Frey, K., & Rivara, F. P. (1997). Effectiveness of a violence prevention curriculum among children in elementary school: A randomized controlled trial. *Journal of the American Medical Association, 277,* 1605–1611.

Harrell, J. S., Gansky, S. A., McMurray, R. G., Bangdiwala, S. I., Frauman, A. C., & Bradley, C. B. (1998). School-based interventions improve heart health in children with multiple cardiovascular risk factors. *Pediatrics, 102,* 371–380.

Hembree-Kigin, T. L., & McNeil, C. B. (1995). *Parent–child interaction therapy.* New York: Plenum Press.

Hurley, E., Chamberlain, A., Slavin, R. E., & Madden, N. A. (2000). *Effects of Success for All on TAAS Reading: A Texas statewide evaluation.* Baltimore, MD: Johns Hopkins University, Center for Research on the Education of Students Placed at Risk.

Jemmott, J. B., Jemmott, L. S., & Fong, G. T. (1992). Reductions in HIV risk-associated sexual behaviors among black male adolescents: Effects of an AIDS prevention intervention. *American Journal of Public Health, 82,* 372–377.

Jemmott, J. B., Jemmott, L. S., & Fong, G. T. (1998). Abstinence and safer sex: HIV risk-reduction interventions for African American adolescents. *Journal of the American Medical Association, 279,* 1529–1536.

Juel, C. (1988). Learning to read and write: A longitudinal study of 54 children from first through fourth grades. *Journal of Educational Psychology, 80,* 437–447.

Kelleher, K. J., Childs, G. E., Wasserman, R. C., McInerney, T. K., Nutting, P. A., & Gardner, W. P. (1997). Insurance status and recognition of psychosocial problems: A report from PROS and ASPN. *Archives of Pediatrics and Adolescent Medicine, 151,* 1109–1115.

Kikano, G. E., Stange, K. C., Flocke, S. A., & Zyzanski, S. J. (1997). Put Prevention into Practice: Outcomes in a family practice center. *Journal of Preventive Medicine, 17,* 73–78.

Lewis, T. J., Sugai, G., & Colvin, G. (1998). Reducing problem behavior through a school-wide system of effective behavioral support: Investigation of a school-wide social skills training program and contextual interventions. *School Psychology Review, 27,* 446–459.

Luepker, R. V., Perry, C. L., McKinlay, S. M., Nader, P. R., Parcel, G. S., Stone, E. J., Webber, L. S., Elder, J. P., Feldman, H. A., Johnson, C. C., Kelder, S. H., & Wu, M. (1996). Outcomes of a field trial to improve children's dietary patterns and physical activity: The Child and Adolescent Trial for Cardiovascular Health (CATCH). *Journal of the American Medical Association, 275,* 768–776.

Lwebuga-Mukasa, J., & Dunn-Georgiou, E. (2002). A school-based asthma intervention program in the Buffalo, New York, schools. *Journal of School Health, 72,* 27–32.

Lyon, G. R. (2002). Reading development, reading difficulties, and reading instruction: Educational and public health issues. *Journal of School Psychology, 40,* 3–6.

Lyon, G. R., Alexander, D., & Yaffe, S. (1997). Progress and promise in research in learning disabilities. *Learning Disabilities: A Multidisciplinary Journal, 8,* 1–6.

Maslach, C., & Leiter, M. (1997). *The truth about burnout.* San Francisco: Jossey-Bass.

Masten, A. S., & Coatsworth, J. D. (1998). The development of competence in favorable and unfavorable environments: Lessons from research on successful children. *American Psychologist, 53,* 205–220.

National Center for Educational Statistics. (2001). NAEP 2000 Reading: A report card for the nation and the states. Washington, DC: U.S. Department of Education.

National Reading Panel. (2000). *Teaching children to read: An evidence-based assessment of the scientific research literature on reading and its implications for reading instruction.* Washington, DC: National Institute of Child Health and Human Development.

Payton, J. W., Wardlaw, D. M., Graczyk, P. A., Bloodworth, M. R., Tompsett, C. J., & Weissberg, R. P. (2000). Social and emotional learning: A framework for promoting mental health and reducing risk behavior in children and youth. *Journal of School Health, 70,* 179–185.

Pianta, R. C. (1999). *Enhancing relationships between children and teachers.* Washington, DC: American Psychological Association.

Power, T. J., & Blom-Hoffman, J. (in press). The school as venue for managing and preventing health problems: Opportunities and challenges. In R. T. Brown (Ed.), *The handbook of pediatric psychology in school settings.* Mahwah, NJ: Erlbaum.

Sameroff, A. J. (1993). Models of development and developmental risk. In C. H. Zeanah (Ed.), *Handbook of infant mental health* (pp. 3–13). New York: Guilford Press.

Shapiro, E. S. (1996). *Academic skills problems: Direct assessment and intervention* (2nd ed.). New York: Guilford Press.

Slavin, R. E., & Madden, N. A. (2001). *One million children: Success for All.* Thousand Oaks, CA: Corwin.

Slavin, R. E., Madden, N. A., & Wasik, B. A. (1997). *Success for All and Roots & Wings: Summary of research on achievement outcomes.* Baltimore, MD: Johns Hopkins University, Center for Research on the Education of Students Placed at Risk.

Smith, L. J., Ross, S. M., & Casey, J. P. (1994). *Special education analyses for Success for All in four cities.* Memphis, TN: University of Memphis, Center for Research in Education Policy.

Stone, R. (1996). *Core issues in comprehensive community-building initiatives.* Chicago: Chapin Hall Center for Children.

Talley, R. C., & Short, R. J. (1995). *School health: Psychology's role. A report to the nation.* Washington, DC: American Psychological Association.

Torgesen, J. K. (2002). The prevention of reading difficulties. *Journal of School Psychology, 40,* 7–26.

Tucker, C. M. (2002). Expanding pediatric psychology beyond hospital wall to meet the health care needs of ethnic minority children. *Journal of Pediatric Psychology, 27,* 315–324.

U.S. Department of Education. (1997). *21st Century Community Learning Centers program.* Washington, DC: Author.

Wahler, R. G., & Dumas, J. E. (1989). Attentional problems in dysfunctional mother–child interactions: An interbehavioral model. *American Psychologist, 105,* 116–130.

CHAPTER 9

Evaluating Programs
of Prevention

The need to design and implement effective programs of prevention has been clearly established. Unfortunately, the effectiveness of many prevention programs has not been examined empirically. In this chapter, we contend that it is critical that program evaluation studies be conducted to establish prevention outcomes in terms of statistical significance, clinical significance, social validity, and cost-effectiveness. First, a rationale for conducting program evaluation is explicated. Second, we delineate several different types of program evaluation designed to answer key questions regarding process and outcome. Third, the advantages and limitations of the most prominent experimental designs used in program evaluation are discussed. As part of this discussion, relatively new methods for longitudinal data analysis are described. Examples of prevention program evaluations are presented to highlight key concepts. Finally, we offer recommendations for evaluating programs of prevention that are implemented in school and pediatric care settings.

RATIONALE FOR PROGRAM EVALUATION

There are many compelling reasons why objective evaluation procedures should be used whenever programs of prevention are implemented in applied settings. (See Table 9.1 for a description of key concepts in evaluation.) Chief among these reasons is the need to ensure that the program produces the intended effects to a significant degree. Ideally, the program's *efficacy* is established through demonstrating its ability to produce the necessary or desired results under controlled experimental conditions. Typically, efficacy studies are conducted in health or education

191

TABLE 9.1. Key Concepts in Program Evaluation

Concept	Definition
Efficacy	Establishing effects of prevention program under controlled experimental conditions.
Effectiveness	Establishing effects of prevention program under "real-world" conditions in applied settings.
Cost-effectiveness	Evaluation that takes into account the costs of conducting a program (including time, resources, and personnel) and the resultant benefits (behavior change and improvements to child, family, and community).
Integrity	Degree to which the prevention program is implemented as intended.
Social validity	Degree to which the prevention program makes a meaningful impact on people's lives.
Accessibility	Degree to which the prevention program is available and considered "user-friendly" by community members.

settings that are part of, or affiliated with, university or research centers. As such, program components are implemented by highly trained staff under the direct supervision of research staff. Although these studies may have strong internal validity, the generalizability of obtained results to "real-world" conditions (i.e., external validity) often is suspect. It is perhaps more important to determine a prevention program's *effectiveness* through examining outcomes under existing conditions in community-based settings. Effectiveness studies are conducted to examine program components that are implemented by individuals employed in schools and healthcare settings in the community. Often, strict adherence to procedures preserving internal validity is sacrificed to ensure that program effects can be generalized to communities for which the program is intended. In addition to establishing that a prevention program works as intended, it is critical to determine whether the program also is cost-efficient. Data regarding cost-effectiveness are particularly compelling when attempting to "sell" the public and/or key policymakers on the need to implement a specific program of prevention. A comparison of costs associated with program utilization and those costs elicited by *not implementing* the prevention program is necessary to make the case for long-term prevention efforts. Given the long-term nature of most prevention efforts, often, this requires estimates of costs incurred over long time periods, which may prove challenging.

Program evaluation can be very helpful in identifying prevention components to retain or discard. Furthermore, data can be used to shape and fine-tune specific procedures in an effort to enhance effectiveness and cost-efficiency. For example, an evaluation study might indicate that prevention effects are primarily elicited through classroom- rather than home-based procedures. Thus, successive iterations of the prevention program might be streamlined by including only those classroom-based strategies that were previously found effective.

Program evaluation provides a critical opportunity to include community members (e.g., parents, teachers, and students) in the design and implementation of the prevention program. Because assessment of program outcomes typically requires multiple methods and informants, a natural linkage among systems can be fostered. For example, Nastasi and colleagues (2000) describe a participatory intervention model (PIM) that provides a mechanism for involving stakeholders in the planning and evaluation of intervention programs. The PIM has been used successfully in designing and implementing programs for reducing sexual risk in several countries and cultures (see Nastasi et al., 2000). Thus, one selling point of program evaluation is that, if done in a participatory manner, one can empower community members and promote their involvement in the prevention program. Fostering empowerment and a sense of inclusion is particularly critical when the prevention program is focused on children from diverse backgrounds (Roosa, Dumka, Gonzales, & Knight, 2002). The acceptability of prevention programs by community members is likely to be enhanced in the context of the participatory model as well (Nastasi et al., 2000). A final, related reason for program evaluation is to establish the social validity of prevention outcomes. Specifically, the prevention scientist must identify the degree to which community stakeholders (e.g., parents, teachers, healthcare professionals, and children) value the program's goals, methods, and results. For example, consumer satisfaction ratings could be obtained from participants before, during, and/or after prevention efforts are implemented. In indicated prevention programs, in which the focus is on reducing health risk, it also may be important to establish social validity of program outcomes by demonstrating that target individuals are "normalized." Stated differently, although statistical significance is important, it is perhaps more important to establish that clinically significant outcomes are obtained through making a meaningful difference in people's lives. One way to study clinical significance is by comparing outcomes of at-risk individuals participating in the prevention program and those associated with typically developing individuals from similar backgrounds.

TYPES OF PROGRAM EVALUATION

Programs of prevention can be evaluated on a variety of levels. Specifically, there are at least five critical questions that can be answered about any proposed program. First, did the program get delivered, and how was it delivered? This question addresses factors related to the process of the program. Second, how well did the program get delivered (i.e., was it delivered as designed)? Treatment integrity is the focus of this evaluation question. Third, what effects did the program have on key assessment measures? This is the most complex and, arguably, the most important question to answer, because it addresses the program's purpose and goals (i.e., effect on outcomes of participants). The next question—What value did the program have for key stakeholders in the community?—focuses on the social validity and acceptability of the prevention program. Finally, what was the significance of the outcomes for the community? This last question addresses the overall impact of the prevention program on the community from a broader perspective.

Process (Did the Program Get Delivered?)

The first step in evaluating a prevention program is to determine whether the program was actually delivered to the intended population. Stated differently, the process of program implementation must be assessed. In order to answer process questions, basic data regarding program participants and frequency of implementation need to be gathered. Specifically, inclusion and exclusion criteria for participants should be established prior to program implementation, and the degree to which actual participants met these criteria should be determined. These data are critical in evaluating whether the program was delivered to the intended population. Next, a record should be kept as to when program sessions were conducted, the length of each session, which participants attended which sessions, and whether program materials were used (e.g., handouts provided to participants). If more detailed process information is needed, then sessions could be audio- or videotaped for later transcription and analysis. For example, one could examine the nature and quality of interactions between session leaders and participants and/or among the participants themselves.

Integrity (How Well Did the Program Get Delivered?)

From an evaluation perspective, the prevention program is the independent variable, and one must determine if the independent variable was manipulated as intended. Thus, whenever possible, data should be collected to determine how well the program was delivered. There are several options for assessing treatment integrity, including direct observation of program implementation, completion of integrity checklists, and examination of permanent products generated by use of the program. Each of these assessment options is reviewed briefly here. Readers interested in a more extensive discussion of treatment integrity assessment can refer to Ehrhardt, Barnett, Lentz, Stollar, and Reifin (1996).

The most direct assessment of intervention integrity is for the evaluator (or someone in the community setting, such as a classroom aide) to observe the implementation of the prevention program on a periodic basis. For example, the evaluator could attend 20% of violence prevention sessions being implemented by a school counselor. During the observation, the evaluator could use a checklist to determine how many of the prescribed program steps were completed as designed (for an example of such a checklist, see Figure 9.1). Thus, one could generate at least two percentages: (1) percentage of program steps implemented correctly and (2) percentage of sessions in which individual components are completed

Violence Prevention Program
Session Integrity Checklist

STEP	COMPLETED	NOT COMPLETED
1. Review homework from last session.		
2. Explain purpose and activities for session.		
3. Show video vignettes in correct sequence.		
4. Lead discussion for at least 5 minutes following each vignette.		
5. Demonstrate strategy to be practiced by participants.		
6. Facilitate role play of strategy by all participants.		
7. Provide feedback to participants following each role play.		
8. Lead participants in discussion of situations when they will use this strategy.		
9. Assign homework to be completed prior to next session.		
10. Summarize main ideas and strategies discussed in session.		

FIGURE 9.1. Intervention integrity checklist for a Violence Prevention Program session.

accurately. The former percentage portrays the overall fidelity of the program and should average at least 90%. The individual component percentage provides the evaluator with critical information regarding which program steps are being completed accurately, and which steps are being missed consistently. The latter information can lead to retraining and/or prompting of missing components, while allowing for specific, positive feedback to the implementer regarding those steps that are used correctly. Typically, it is difficult to conduct observations of treatment integrity on more than an occasional basis. Under these conditions, it is possible that implementation integrity may differ across sessions depending on the presence or absence of an observer (i.e., reactivity effect). For these reasons, the person implementing the prevention program (e.g., teacher, counselor, or psychologist) could be asked to complete an integrity checklist during and/or following *every* intervention session that would list the prevention program steps in a similar or even identical fashion to the form used by an observer, as discussed earlier. Although self-report checklists of intervention integrity might be subject to bias, these could provide the same information as observations, including the percentage of steps implemented correctly and the degree to which individual program components are completed accurately across sessions. Another option is to audio- or videotape every program session and randomly select tapes for integrity checks (Power, Dowrick, Ginsburg-Block, & Manz, 2002). Presumably, program leaders will endeavor to maintain high levels of implementation accuracy, because they do not know which sessions will be evaluated for integrity.

Some prevention programs involve the completion of tasks by the implementer and/or participants that generate permanent products. For example, violence prevention sessions might include brainstorming exercises wherein participants develop a written list of ideas on how to handle conflict situations. Permanent products can be collected for later inspection by the evaluator, who can determine whether program components have been completed as intended based on session outcomes. Ideally, program integrity would be evaluated using all three indices (observations, self-report checklists, and permanent products) to provide as comprehensive a picture as possible of the degree to which prevention strategies are being implemented as intended. This is valuable information not only for evaluation purposes but also to provide program implementers with feedback about how well they are using the program, along with suggestions on how implementation could be improved. In order to achieve the latter, treatment integrity data should be shared with program implementers on an ongoing basis.

One problem with most conventional methods for assessing treatment integrity is that they focus almost exclusively on the content of the prevention or intervention program, while neglecting important process issues. Specifically, the relationship between program participants and individuals implementing the prevention program (e.g., teachers, healthcare professionals, or school psychologists) often is critical to program success. Thus, methods to assess interactions among participants and other process variables should be included, whenever possible, when monitoring program integrity. For example, audiotapes of prevention sessions could be transcribed and analyzed to identify key positive and negative verbal interactions among participants. Another alternative would be to interview selected child participants periodically during the prevention program to ascertain perceptions of relationships with the program leader or other participating children.

Outcome (What Effects Did the Program Have on Target Skills or Behaviors?)

One of the most important areas for program evaluation is to assess the degree to which intended outcomes (i.e., program goals) are achieved. Program effects on key dependent measures go a long way in determining whether the specific prevention strategies should be used in the future. There are several critical decisions that a program evaluator must make in assessing outcomes. First, the specific dependent measures must be chosen that tap behaviors and constructs reflective of program goals. Ideally, measures will incorporate the perspectives of multiple informants and include a variety of assessment techniques. Second, the experimental design needs to be selected. A balance between internal and external validity concerns should be achieved. Finally, the evaluator must choose how the data will be analyzed using descriptive and/or inferential statistics.

Typically, prevention programs can have at least two goals: (1) reduction in the frequency of potential negative outcomes and (2) improvement in key areas of functioning (e.g., academic and social competence). Thus, the evaluation protocol should include measures that reflect both possible goal areas (McConaughy & Leone, 2001). Measures could include teacher and/or parent behavior rating scales, direct observations of behavior in key environments (e.g., classroom and playground; Nolan & Gadow, 1994), as well as archival data (e.g., school records of disciplinary referrals and report card grades). Standardized measures such as academic achievement tests also might be included, depending on the focus of the prevention program.

There are several critical considerations for selecting outcome measures for a specific program evaluation (for review, see McConaughy & Leone, 2001). First, measures should be psychometrically sound (i.e., adequate reliability and validity) and measure the construct targeted by the prevention program as closely as possible. For example, if a program is oriented toward preventing antisocial behavior, then outcome measures must have adequate construct and criterion-related validity as indices of aggression, disruption, and other antisocial acts. Second, the perspectives and judgments of multiple informants should be included, particularly those of key stakeholders (e.g., parents, teachers, and the students themselves). In similar fashion, the evaluation should not rely on a single assessment mode (e.g., behavior rating scales) and, ideally, would include multiple methods. The use of multiple methods and informants acknowledges the fact that in program evaluation, there is rarely a "gold standard" for assessing outcome; therefore, the limitations of each method can be counterbalanced by the strengths of another index.

When programs are implemented for children from diverse backgrounds, assessment measures must be sensitive to this diversity, especially in the context of how this diversity impacts child functioning at the local level (Roosa et al., 2002). Furthermore, the measurement equivalence of assessment indices should be established (Knight & Hill, 1998). Specifically, one must determine whether a measure examines the same construct in an equivalent fashion across cultural and ethnic groups, especially for those groups represented in the prevention program (Reid et al., 1998). A final consideration in selecting evaluation measures is their relative cost-effectiveness and the feasibility of obtaining data. When resources are limited, evaluations will need to be done with a minimum number of critical measures that assess the primary targets as closely as possible. Also, the least expensive way to collect data should be determined. For example, paraprofessionals might be recruited to conduct behavior observations as an alternative to more costly options (e.g., school counselors or school psychologists).

Outcome evaluation should include explicit a priori decisions regarding the experimental design that will be used. Later in this chapter, we provide examples of group and single-subject designs that could be used for program evaluation. There is no right or wrong choice with respect to design; rather, one must balance needs for internal and external validity, as well as consider feasibility in making this decision. Our main point is that *some type* of experimental design must be used, and this decision should be made before the prevention program is implemented. Similarly, one must consider options for statistical analysis and make decisions up front as to how outcome data will be analyzed. Typically, data are evaluated with both descriptive and inferential statistics (for review, see McConaughy & Leone, 2001). Regardless of the specific statistical procedure employed, it is important to go beyond a simple consideration of statistical significance and include measures that characterize the magnitude of prevention effect (e.g., effect size; see Cohen, 1992). Specific options for statistical analysis are delineated later in the chapter.

Social Validity (What Value Did the Program Have for the Community?)

The degree to which community stakeholders value the prevention program is assumed to have a direct impact on how likely program components will actually be used in the future (i.e., treatment acceptability is highly related to treatment integrity; Reimers, Wacker, & Koeppl, 1987). Although acceptability of the program is presumed to be related to its success or failure (i.e., program outcomes), other factors may be equally important to consider, such as the feasibility of implementation; costs, financial and otherwise, associated with using the program; and the degree to which program and community values are consonant.

Program acceptability can be assessed through interviews with representative stakeholders, including teachers, parents, students, and related services personnel. Care should be taken to get a "representative sample" given that time constraints typically preclude interviewing all participants. Whenever possible, interviews should be conducted by someone who does not have a direct investment in the program (e.g., school principal). Interviews should include questions regarding satisfaction with the process and outcomes of the program, as well as the costs associated with its implementation. Cost considerations should extend beyond monetary resources and also assess the degree to which personnel, time, and effort were expended. Stakeholders should report whether they believe that program benefits outweighed the costs. Participants should be asked whether they would complete the program again, if given the choice, as well as whether they would recommend the program to their peers. Suggestions for modifications to the program should be solicited as well.

When time does not permit interviews to be conducted, stakeholders might be asked to complete consumer satisfaction or treatment acceptability checklists. A variety of acceptability measures have been developed specifically to examine satisfaction with psychological consultation (Sheridan & Steck, 1995) and behavioral interventions (Witt & Elliott, 1985). These measures might be adapted to reflect specific components of prevention programs. Again, it is best for these measures to be completed outside of the presence of program implementers or others who have a direct investment in program outcomes (to avoid the potential of biasing the consumer report). In fact, anonymous ratings would be preferred to circumvent the potential for biased reports. Although acceptability checklists primarily include forced-choice items using Likert scales, these items should be supplemented with open-ended questions soliciting suggestions for program modification.

Historically, intervention acceptability has been assessed only at the completion of a prevention program; however, evaluators should consider getting acceptability data on a more ongoing basis (Reimers, Wacker, Cooper, & DeRaad, 1992). Our premise is that community stakeholders need to be involved in the design and planning of prevention programs for the latter to be most successful. Thus, it would be important to evaluate program acceptability *before*, *during*, and *after* prevention strategies are used. These data could then be used to fine-tune program components to meet best the values and needs of community stakeholders.

Impact (What Was the Significance of the Outcomes for the Community?)

Beyond consideration of the effects and acceptability of a prevention program, it also is important to determine what significance the program has had for the community and for key stakeholders. Several questions are pertinent to the evaluation of a program's impact. First, to what degree did the program result in clinically significant outcomes for participants and affiliated community members? Determination of statistical significance is not sufficient in establishing that clinically important and relevant effects have been obtained (Kazdin, 2000). There are a number of ways in which clinical significance can be assessed (see Kazdin, 1999). For example, one could ascertain the degree to which the prevention program brings the outcomes of an at-risk sample into the normal range (Kendall, Marrs-Garcia, Nath, & Sheldrick, 1999). Stated differently, do children who participated in the prevention program "look like" their normal peers over the short- and long-term with respect to the behaviors or outcomes of interest (i.e., has normalization occurred)? The impact of prevention programs can also be determined by assessing variables known to be associated with good health, such as a balanced diet, regular exercise, weight within the normal range, good attendance in school, peer acceptance, a strong attachment with a caregiver, and family involvement in education.

Another method for assessing clinical significance is to ask key stakeholders (e.g., teachers and parents) to provide subjective evaluations of the degree to which the prevention program has made a difference in participants' lives. This line of questioning goes beyond simple acceptability of the program, which has to do with feasibility, availability of resources, and other pragmatic issues. In terms of impact, it is important to assess whether the program has made a measurable difference in the lives of participating children, in the eyes of those who live and work with them every day.

A final method for evaluating clinical significance is to document social impact by considering how the program has affected the child's functioning in ways that are important to teachers, parents, and other community members (Drotar, 2002). The latter would require inclusion of dependent measures that go beyond assessment of the primary outcome constructs. For example, the social impact of a drug prevention program could be evaluated by using teacher or parent questionnaires regarding children's social skills.

A second question related to a program's impact is to what degree did the program improve the lives of community members over the long term? This assessment would extend beyond measurement of long-term effects on the primary targets of the program (see earlier Outcome section). For example, one could calculate the monetary and person-hour costs of the prevention program relative to costs associated with negative outcomes that the program is intended to prevent (e.g., incarceration, institutionalization, and enrollment in substance abuse programs). To the extent that the prevention program reduces the latter costs, economic benefits may accrue to the community as a function of prevention efforts.

A third question related to impact is whether the prevention program continues to be sought after and used by community members over the long term (i.e., sustainability). Sustainability refers to the extent to which the program can maintain itself after funding ends or the period of intensive planning and evaluation is over. Sustainability is related to the degree to which community stakeholders are committed to the program and assume ownership for the initiative. In order for a community to make a long-term commitment to a program, the latter must not only be acceptable but also must be perceived as making a meaningful difference in people's lives. Thus, a program evaluator could track the number of years that a program is in operation, as well as the degree of demand for the program (e.g., numbers of children referred and frequency of program implementation per calendar year) within a given community.

EXPERIMENTAL DESIGN AND DATA ANALYSIS OPTIONS

One of the most important decisions in evaluating programs of prevention is selecting an experimental design that will isolate program-induced effects. Once data are collected, one also must choose how to analyze the results such that evaluation and research questions are answered in an optimal fashion. In this section, we briefly describe the most common experimental methods that researchers and practitioners can use for program evaluation. Design choices include those that are experimentally controlled (e.g., randomized control group) and those that involve less experimental control of threats to internal validity (e.g., quasi-experimental designs). Experimental designs also may differ between those that involve aggregation of group-level data and those that include continuous measurement of one or more single participants or units of study (i.e., single-subject designs). Data derived from a program evaluation typically are analyzed with traditional statistical procedures (e.g., repeated measures analysis of variance). The use and limitations of these statistical analyses are described (see Table 9.2). Recently, prevention and intervention researchers have used relatively novel statistical procedures (e.g., hierarchical linear modeling) to circumvent limitations and to portray outcomes more comprehensively.

TABLE 9.2. Advantages and Limitations of Various Evaluation Designs

Type of design	Advantages	Limitations
Randomized control group	Controls for threats to internal validity.	May be unfeasible or unethical.
	Results can be generalized to population.	Requires large sample.
		Lacks individualized treatment.
	Inferential statistics can be used.	
Quasi-experimental group	More feasible than randomized design.	Incomplete control of threats to validity.
	Results can be generalized to population.	Requires large sample.
		Lacks individualized treatment.
	Inferential statistics can be used.	
ABA or reversal design (single subject)	Control for threats to internal validity.	May be unfeasible or unethical.
	Can evaluate effects on level and trend of outcomes.	Limited external validity.
		Prevention effects are not "reversible."
Multiple baseline (single subject)	Control for threats to internal validity.	Limited external validity.
	Can evaluate effects on level and trend of outcomes.	May be unfeasible.

Group Experimental and Quasi-Experimental Designs

The optimal experimental design for controlling potential threats to internal validity is the pre–post randomized control group study. Participants are randomly assigned to the intervention (or in this case, *prevention*) and control groups prior to initial data collection. Dependent measures are collected prior to and following implementation of the program. In the case of prevention evaluation, data also should be collected after an appropriate follow-up period. Because participants are randomly assigned to groups, typical threats to internal validity (e.g., history, maturation, and selection bias) are controlled, assuming that a sufficient-size sample is used (Kazdin, 2000). Furthermore, the use of a control group that does not receive the prevention program allows one to determine whether outcomes are related to prevention strategies as opposed to extraneous variables typically associated with maturation and/or development over time. Variations of this experimental design can include (1) the use of attention or wait-list control rather than no-treatment control groups, (2) evaluation of two or more prevention programs simultaneously in a multigroup design, and (3) multiple data collection points over time to determine time-dependent programmatic effects. The specific components of the design should be selected on the basis of how best to answer the research question(s).

Although the randomized control group design is ideal with respect to controlling for threats to internal validity, there are important limitations to this design option, particularly for use in applied settings. Specifically, the prevention researcher or clinician rarely has the opportunity or authority to assign children randomly to classroom or therapeutic settings. Also, the use of a control group (especially a no-treatment control group) may be questioned by community members based on ethical grounds. The external validity or degree to which results can be generalized to "real-world" conditions also is suspect given that this degree of experimental control rarely is seen under typical conditions in the community.

Because of the inherent limitations of the "true" experimental design, applied social researchers have sought alternatives that can control for some but not all threats to internal validity. These alternatives or quasi-experimental designs also have the advantage of being more feasible for use in community settings (Cook & Campbell, 1979). For example, one could evaluate outcomes in the context of a single group (which receives the prevention program), wherein measures are collected prior to and following program implementation. Of course, this single-group design is subject to myriad potential threats to internal validity. A better option would be to include two or more groups, each of which is evaluated pre- and postintervention; one group receives the prevention program, and the others receive an alternative program or no program. Because participants are not randomly assigned to groups (but rather are assigned based on decisions made by the school or agency), this is not a "true" experiment. Nevertheless, some threats to internal validity (e.g., maturation) are controlled for by this design. Additional examples of quasi-experimental designs for use in applied settings can be obtained by consulting Cook and Campbell (1979).

Single-Subject Designs

In many evaluation situations, the prevention researcher or clinician is interested in outcomes for individual participants or units (e.g., students, classrooms, schools, or neighborhoods). In such cases, a single-subject rather than a group design may be used. Single-subject designs have a long history of use in the fields of experimental analysis of behavior and applied behavior analysis (Hersen & Barlow, 1982; Johnston & Pennypacker, 1980; Kazdin, 1992). Typically, these designs involve the collection of one or more dependent measures on a continuous basis across days, weeks, or longer time periods. At a minimum, there are two conditions to the evaluation, including baseline (measurement prior to the prevention program being implemented) and intervention. Design options such as the reversal or withdrawal design and the multiple baseline design are considered "true" experiments in that they can control for threats to internal validity and allow the researcher to attribute causality to the independent variable (i.e., prevention program). There also are options for evaluating the differential effects of two or more programs (e.g., alternating treatment design).

As is the case for the randomized control group design, it may be difficult to implement controlled single-subject designs in applied settings. For example, teachers or parents may object to a reversal design, because they have ethical concerns with the removal of an effective intervention (i.e., to establish a return to baseline). Thus, practitioners may choose to use controlled case study designs that involve only two conditions (i.e., baseline and treatment; Kazdin, 1992). If the case study includes certain key features such as continuous collection of objective data and experimenter-determined phase changes, then more confidence can be attributed to the results (Bergan & Kratochwill, 1990; Kazdin, 1992). Thus, the controlled case study option is similar to quasi-experimental designs that were discussed for group-level evaluations.

Data collected in the context of a single-subject design can be analyzed in several ways (Hersen & Barlow, 1982; Kazdin, 1992). First, the evaluator may calculate changes in the mean or the level across phases.

Consideration of change in level is similar to analysis of pre–post mean differences in a group design. Second, one of the advantages of a single-subject relative to a group design is that the former allows consideration of other possible changes in dependent measures. Thus, changes in trend can be examined by calculating data slopes within each phase, then making comparisons across phases. Changes in trend may be particularly important in the evaluation of prevention programs, because programmatic effects could involve a slowing of the development of a problematic behavior (e.g., frequency of alcohol use) over time relative to control conditions. A third focus of data analysis would be to determine changes in intercept across conditions. Specifically, one would compare the last data point in the baseline condition with the first data point in the prevention condition. This difference would represent the latency or immediacy of the treatment effect. Typically, latency is less critical for prevention programs wherein change over the long term is of greatest interest. An analysis of change in variability across phases sheds light on the consistency of participant performance over time. The range of data points within each condition is calculated, wherein the difference in ranges across phases indicates the degree to which the prevention program enhances or detracts from behavioral consistency. Additional statistical analyses are possible in the context of single-subject designs (for review, see Kazdin, 1992); however, the visual analytic methods, described earlier, typically are sufficient in characterizing evaluation outcomes.

Single-subject designs offer clear advantages relative to group designs in that the former allow for a more comprehensive picture of program effects on individual participants or target units. In group designs, one typically examines differences in means across groups and/or experimental conditions. Although consideration of group means offers a "snapshot" of programmatic effects on the overall group, the generality of prevention outcomes to individual participants is suspect (i.e., the group mean may not represent the effect for some or even many of the participants). In contrast, the continuous data available in a single-subject design can provide details regarding changes not only in mean performance but also with respect to alterations in the trajectory of outcome data over time. In fact, the advantages of single-subject designs have been touted as an impetus for practitioners and researchers working in applied settings to use these designs more frequently than group options (Hayes, 1981).

Alternatively, there are several limitations of single-subject designs for prevention research. Because data are collected on a small number of participants or units, the generalizability of obtained results to the population of similar individuals or units is questionable. Generalizability to the population is one important element of external validity. Another disadvantage is that continuous data collection may be impractical or impossible in some community settings with limited resources. In similar fashion, if the prevention program is focused on long-term outcomes (e.g., reduction in HIV infection or risk of heart disease), continuous data collection over time is not an option. Another limitation is that the ABA reversal design is particularly ill-suited to prevention research, especially when the latter is focused on long- rather than short-term outcomes. Thus, the selection of a single-subject design must be done carefully, while considering inherent advantages and limitations of these designs, as well as the degree to which evaluation questions are addressed by the specific design selected.

Statistical Analyses of Program Outcomes

Evaluations involving the collection of group-level data typically are followed by an analysis of the statistical significance of obtained effects. Most frequently, a univariate or multivariate analysis of variance (ANOVA) is used to establish whether groups differ in mean outcomes as a function of prevention efforts. More specifically, a mixed-model ANOVA is used that includes one or more between-groups factors (e.g., prevention vs. control group) and a within-group, repeated-measures factor (pre- vs. post-treatment). The statistical significance of the resultant F ratio is determined and post hoc tests (e.g., Scheffé) are used to isolate where specific between-group differences may occur (e.g., at postintervention rather than at preintervention).

An exclusive reliance on null hypothesis significance testing has been criticized, because determination of statistical significance provides limited information about outcomes (Cohen, 1994). Specifically, results that are statistically significant merely indicate that the likelihood of the null hypothesis (i.e., no differences between groups and/or assessment phases) being true is low. As a result, the clinical significance of obtained findings is more important to determine. For example, one could calculate an effect size (Cohen, 1992) to represent the magnitude of differences between groups. Becker (1988) has proposed an effect size that captures the magnitude of change over time in a treatment group relative to change exhibited by a control group over the same time period. The latter effect size, referred to as a Δ, is particularly appropriate for calculating the size of prevention program effects. Another option for determining the clinical significance of program effects is to calculate a reliable change index (Jacobsen & Truax, 1991), which indicates the degree that change over time exceeds the standard error of measurement of a specific dependent measure. If normative data are available, one also can determine the extent to which the prevention program brings an at-risk group into the normal range (another important facet of clinical significance).

Although the ANOVA and similar analytic procedures have helped to advance prevention science, several properties of these techniques limit their utility. First, ANOVA models typically examine between-group and/or between-phase changes in level or mean only. Consideration of more complex models of change (e.g., curvilinear function) is difficult and unwieldy. Given that prevention programs are intended to alter trajectories of key behaviors, this is a critical limitation of the ANOVA approach. Second, ANOVA models do not examine individual differences in change over time. Stated differently, the ANOVA approach models change at the group level only; thereby losing important information regarding the degree to which prevention program effects vary across individuals. Finally, if a participant is missing as little as one data point, then all of that participant's data cannot be used for any analyses on that variable. Depending on the degree of missing data, a significant percentage of participants can be "lost," thereby deleteriously affecting the power and generalizability of the data analyses. Because evaluations of prevention programs often involve collection of data over long time periods, missing data are a frequent occurrence. Thus, traditional analyses such as ANOVA and multivariate analyses of variance (MANOVA) can be quite limited for modeling prevention program outcomes.

In recent years, several alternative data-analytic strategies have been used to circumvent the limitations of "traditional" analyses. Hierarchical linear modeling (HLM) or multilevel analysis involves explicit modeling of both intercept (i.e., mean) and slope (i.e., trajectory) indices at two or more levels (Bryk & Raudenbush, 1992). Typically, a researcher will propose models for change at both individual and group (e.g., classroom or school) levels based on theory and/or the results of prior empirical studies. Thus, program effects can be characterized by changes in trajectory and level at individual and group levels. Furthermore, nonlinear change models (e.g., quadratic) can be examined quite readily. HLM analyses incorporate all available data, including data from participants who have missed one or more assessment phases, thereby providing as complete a picture as possible of program effects. Despite the clear advantages of HLM over the traditional ANOVA approach, HLM requires relatively large samples, and the robustness of these techniques when assumptions are violated is relatively unknown (Bryk & Raudenbush, 1992).

Second-generation structural equation modeling (SEM) procedures can be used to model change resulting from a prevention program. Muthén (2001) has proposed SEM procedures that can include both categorical (e.g., group membership) and continuous (e.g., behavioral construct) variables examined over time. Although complex, this SEM approach could provide a comprehensive picture of prevention program effects. As is the case for HLM, however, the SEM approach requires large samples to provide statistically reliable results. Furthermore, the complexities of this statistical technique may be beyond the skills of many prevention researchers or practitioners, thus necessitating additional training (see Klem, 2000).

Many times, the goal of a prevention program is to reduce the probability of one or more events from occurring (e.g., onset of alcohol or tobacco use, becoming pregnant, or perpetration of a violent act). Procedures such as ANOVA, HLM, or SEM are inappropriate to evaluate the extent to which a program prevents a one-time or discrete event. Survival analysis, which has a long history of use in the medical field, can be used to answer questions about event occurrence over long time periods (Willett & Singer, 1993). In discrete-time survival analysis, a sample hazard function can be calculated to indicate the proportion of participants who experience the event over a specified period of time. Furthermore, the hazard function can be used to calculate the probability of event occurrence among remaining participants within prevention and control groups. Thus, one is able to characterize prevention program outcomes in terms of risk probabilities relative to a control condition. For example, one could calculate the probability of adolescents engaging in substance abuse as a function of participating in drug prevention programs in high school. Survival analysis has many advantages (e.g., minimal assumptions and ease of analysis) for use in prevention program evaluations, so long as a discrete event is the primary outcome variable.

Regardless of the statistical analysis conducted, several factors need to be considered when conducting long-term program evaluations. First, one must estimate and account for missing data and/or participant attrition. As mentioned earlier, missing data may require removal of cases from the data set if an ANOVA approach is used. Several methods for modeling missing data and imputing values for key variables have been developed for use in SEM and HLM (for reviews, see Graham, Taylor, & Cumsille, 2001; Schafer, 2001). Also, power analyses (Cohen, 1992) should be conducted beforehand to determine the necessary sample size, *while taking into account potential attrition* estimated from prior empirical investigations and/or implementation of similar programs. Stated differently, one must deal with missing data and participant attrition proactively, because these events are inevitable in a longitudinal design.

A second factor that can have an impact on prevention program evaluation is limited financial and personnel resources to investigate program outcomes. Programs implemented in community settings under typical conditions, with no grant support, are particularly prone to limited resources. One alternative to consider is the use of a cohort-sequential or accelerated longitudinal design, wherein a long-term investigation is "simulated" by conducting several short-term evaluations with different age groups simultaneously (Duncan, Duncan, & Hops, 1996). A cohort-sequential design can be used to estimate a common developmental trajectory over an entire age period covered. For example, if one is interested in investigating the development of antisocial behavior over a 10-year span, one can examine this behavior within 5 separate age cohorts, each representing a 2-year interval within the entire 10-year period (e.g., 5–6 years, 7–8 years, 9–10 years, 11–12 years, and 13–14 years).

A final factor that may limit conclusions based on program evaluation is that the latter is conducted in the context of a rapidly changing field. Given that prevention program efforts typically are oriented toward altering long-term outcomes, many changes in the field could occur during the course of the evaluation. At a pragmatic level, assessment measures that are preferred within a given field of study may change over time, thus rendering the results of a long-term evaluation somewhat obsolete. From a theoretical perspective, a field of study may experience shifts in how key constructs are conceptualized and measured. Once again, if paradigm shifts occur, the results of a long-term evaluation could become moot. Although there is no way to predict and account for shifts within a field of study, one must attempt to include measures and constructs that are likely to stand the test of time, especially if an evaluation is being conducted over a period of several years.

EXAMPLES OF PREVENTION PROGRAM EVALUATIONS

To clarify some of the concepts reviewed in this chapter, we briefly review three examples of prevention program evaluations. Examples include a program with relatively positive outcomes (i.e., Fast Track), a program with mixed outcomes (Every Day, Lots of Ways nutrition education), and a program with minimal outcome (Drug Awareness Resistance Education).

Fast Track

The goal of the Fast Track program is to prevent conduct disorders and related antisocial problem behaviors in adolescents (Conduct Problems Prevention Research Group, 1992, 2002). This program includes universal and selected prevention components that have been evaluated empirically in large samples of nonrisk and high-risk elementary school children. Prevention effects for the high-risk sample were evaluated in the context of a multisite, multicomponent protocol wherein participants were randomly assigned to either an intervention or a no-treatment control group (Conduct Problems Prevention Research Group, 1999). Kindergarten children ($n = 891$) identified as high-risk for conduct problems on the basis of exhibiting significant disruptive behavior in the classroom were selected for participation. For the universal component, classroom teachers in grade 1 implemented the Promoting Alternative Thinking Strategies (PATHS) curriculum, which included classwide lessons related to social problem-solving and friendship skills (Bierman, Greenberg, & Conduct Problems Prevention Research Group, 1996). Indicated prevention strategies (administered only with the high-risk sample) included social skills training, academic tutoring, parent training, and home visits. Thus, prevention components were implemented across home and school settings, and involved parent–teacher collaboration throughout the first-grade academic year.

The evaluation included dependent measures assessing multiple areas of functioning that could be affected by the Fast Track program, including child social cognition; reading skills; child peer relations and social competence; parenting behavior and social cognition; and child aggressive–disruptive behavior. Measures were collected at the end of the kindergarten (preintervention) and first-grade (postintervention) school years. Hierarchical linear modeling procedures were used to analyze the evaluation data. Results indicated statistically significant effects in most of the areas targeted by this prevention program, including both child and parent outcomes. For the most part, effect sizes were in the moderate range, with the greatest effects on reducing aggressive behavior at home and school. Parents reported high levels of satisfaction with the program, and nearly 75% of the sample completed at least 50% of the home-based training. These data support the short-term effectiveness of the Fast Track program; however, given the long-term goal of reducing adolescent antisocial behavior, ongoing evaluation will be necessary to determine fully whether these prevention efforts have been successful.

Every Day, Lots of Ways Nutrition Education Curriculum (Mixed Outcome)

Another potential focus of universal prevention programs is to promote healthier lifestyles among children and adolescents. The Every Day, Lots of Ways (EDLW) nutrition education curriculum (Pennsylvania Department of Education, 1996) is designed to promote eating behaviors among elementary school children in Pennsylvania that are consistent with the food pyramid and Federal dietary guidelines (U.S. Department of Health and Human Services, 2000). EDLW is an integrated curriculum wherein nutrition education lessons are taught by general education teachers within the academic curriculum (e.g., math, science, and social studies). Lessons include teacher-led instruction, classroom activities, and homework, along with goal-setting and self-monitoring procedures to encourage greater consumption of fruits and vegetables. The curriculum varies slightly across kindergarten through 6th grade but is consistent in including the aforementioned components.

Blom-Hoffman and DuPaul (2002) evaluated outcomes associated with the EDLW program in an inner-city elementary school with a predominantly African American student body. A pretest–posttest comparison group quasi-experimental design with a 1-month follow-up was used, including dependent measures that assessed knowledge change (e.g., curriculum-based knowledge tests), behavior change (e.g., observations of lunch plate waste), colds and absenteeism, and parent nutrition knowledge. Participants included 103 children in grades kindergarten through 5, who received the EDLW curriculum, and 70 comparison children, who did not receive EDLW. A series of 2 (group) × 3 (time) ANOVA with repeated measures across time was used to analyze the outcome data.

Mixed results were obtained regarding EDLW effects for this sample. On the positive side, statistically significant effects on knowledge change were obtained, wherein children who participated in the EDLW lessons exhibited greater knowledge of nutrition guidelines at posttest than did comparison children. For the most part, EDLW lessons were implemented accurately by classroom teachers and were found to be acceptable to parents, teachers, and students. Alternatively, minimal changes in children's eating behaviors were found. A post hoc analysis indicated that children consistently exposed to behavior change strategies (goal setting and self-monitoring) were more likely to alter eating behavior (i.e., eat more vegetables) than those children whose classroom teachers did not consistently use behavior change techniques. Thus, the short-term (across one school year) effects of the EDLW program appeared to be restricted to knowledge change.

Drug Awareness Resistance Education (Minimal Outcome)

The Drug Awareness Resistance Education (DARE) program was developed by the Los Angeles Police Department and Los Angeles Unified School District in 1983, as a school-based curriculum designed to prevent drug abuse. It is one of the most frequently used substance abuse programs used in U.S. schools. Although this universal prevention program can be used from late elementary school through high school, the most popular and widely studied component is a 17-lesson curriculum delivered to students in the fifth or sixth grades. This core curriculum is taught by a uniformed police officer and consists of classroom-based lectures, group discussions, question-and-answer sessions, audiovisual materials, workbook exercises, and role playing. The goal of the core DARE program is to teach children the skills they need to recognize and resist pressure to use alcohol, tobacco, and illicit drugs.

The effects of the DARE program have been evaluated by several independent investigative teams (for a meta-analysis, see Ringwalt et al., 1994). The best of these evaluations have included short- and long-term assessment of drug use in large samples of participants randomly assigned to DARE and non-DARE classrooms. Univariate and multivariate analyses of variance were used to examine the statistical significance of group differences over time. Other than a few isolated short-term effects on tobacco and alcohol use, DARE and non-DARE children did not differ significantly with respect to drug use. Furthermore, even effect sizes for social skills and attitude toward drug use were small (i.e., < .20; Ringwalt et al., 1994). These weak effects could be explained by the relatively passive teaching methods and the absence of continued instruction geared toward development of social competence (Ringwalt et al., 1994).

CONCLUSIONS AND RECOMMENDATIONS

Prevention program evaluation is a necessity, not a luxury. The collection of evaluation data not only establishes the effectiveness of a program but also provides important information regarding programmatic process, integrity, acceptability, and impact. Thus, the choice is not whether to conduct an evaluation, but rather *how* to conduct an evaluation (i.e., choosing measures, experimental design, and data analysis procedures). These decisions must be made a priori through collaboration with program stakeholders, while balancing scientific needs (e.g., internal and external validity) on the one hand, and feasibility and cost-efficiency on the other.

The following 10 recommendations are offered in an attempt to help clinicians and prevention researchers conduct high-quality evaluations:

1. Include key stakeholders in the design of the program evaluation, and make sure that the design and measures account for ethnic, linguistic, and socioeconomic diversity.
2. Evaluation design should achieve a balance between internal and external validity concerns, as well as feasibility and cost-efficiency.

3. Use psychometrically sound measures that assess intended outcomes as closely as possible.
4. Evaluate all aspects of program (i.e., process, integrity, outcome, acceptability, and impact) to provide a comprehensive picture of prevention efforts.
5. Get multiple perspectives of program outcome by using multiple assessment methods and multiple informants.
6. Consider the use of single-subject designs and/or nontraditional statistical analyses in order to characterize prevention outcomes best.
7. Collect integrity and process data periodically, and use these to provide feedback and reinforcement to program implementers, so that program modifications are based on data.
8. Develop strategies for reducing attrition and missing data, while also planning for how these difficulties will be handled in the data analyses.
9. Go beyond establishing statistical significance of program effects by determining the magnitude and clinical significance of effects.
10. Communicate your findings to all relevant communities (i.e., go beyond publication in scientific journals) to have maximal impact on prevention activities in the "real world." Collaborate with stakeholders to interpret the meaning of evaluation results and to discuss implications for prevention programming in the future.

REFERENCES

Becker, B. J. (1988). Synthesizing standardized mean-change measures. *British Journal of Mathematical and Statistical Psychology, 41*, 257–278.

Bergan, J. R., & Kratochwill, T. R. (1990). *Behavioral consultation and therapy.* New York: Plenum Press.

Bierman, K. L., Greenberg, M. T., & Conduct Problems Prevention Research Group. (1996). Social skills training in the Fast Track program. In R. D. Peters & R. J. McMahon (Eds.), *Preventing childhood disorders, substance abuse, and delinquency* (pp. 65–89). Thousand Oaks, CA: Sage.

Blom-Hoffman, J., & DuPaul, G. J. (2002). *Intervening in dietary habits of African-American children: An impact evaluation of the Every Day, Lots of Ways interdisciplinary nutrition education curriculum.* Manuscript submitted for publication.

Bryk, A., & Raudenbush, S. (1992). *Hierarchical linear models in social and behavioral research: Applications and data analysis methods.* Newbury Park, CA: Sage.

Cohen, J. (1992). A power primer. *Psychological Bulletin, 112,* 155–169.

Cohen, J. (1994). The earth is round (*p* < .05). *American Psychologist, 49,* 997–1003.

Conduct Problems Prevention Research Group. (1992). A developmental and clinical model for the prevention of conduct disorders: The FAST Track program. *Development and Psychopathology, 4,* 509–527.

Conduct Problems Prevention Research Group. (1999). Initial impact of the Fast Track Prevention trial for conduct problems: I. The high-risk sample. *Journal of Consulting and Clinical Psychology, 67,* 631–647.

Conduct Problems Prevention Research Group. (2002). The implementation of the Fast Track program: An example of a large-scale prevention science efficacy trial. *Journal of Abnormal Child Psychology, 30,* 1–18.

Cook, T. D., & Campbell, D. T. (1979). *Quasi-experimentation: Design and analysis issues for field settings.* Boston: Houghton Mifflin.

Drotar, D. (2002). Enhancing reviews of psychological treatments with pediatric populations: Thoughts on next steps. *Journal of Pediatric Psychology, 27,* 167–176.

Duncan, S. C., Duncan, T. E., & Hops, H. (1996). Analysis of longitudinal data within accelerated longitudinal designs. *Psychological Methods, 1,* 236–248.

Ehrhardt, K. E., Barnett, D. W., Lentz, F. E., Stollar, S. A., & Reifin, L. H. (1996). Innovative methodology in ecological consultation: Use of scripts to promote treatment acceptability and integrity. *School Psychology Quarterly, 11,* 149–168.

Graham, J. W., Taylor, B. J., & Cumsille, P. E. (2001). Planned missing-data designs in analysis of change. In L. M. Collins & A. G. Sayer (Eds.), *New methods for the analysis of change* (pp. 333–354). Washington, DC: American Psychological Association.

Hayes, S. C. (1981). Single case experimental design and empirical clinical practice. *Journal of Consulting and Clinical Psychology, 49,* 193–211.

Hersen, M., & Barlow, D. H. (1982). *Single case experimental designs: Strategies for studying behavior change.* Elmsford, NY: Pergamon Press.

Jacobsen, N. S., & Truax, P. (1991). Clinical significance: A statistical approach to defining meaningful change in psychotherapy research. *Journal of Consulting and Clinical Psychology, 59,* 12–19.

Johnston, J. M., & Pennypacker, H. S. (1980). *Strategies and tactics of human behavioral research.* Hillsdale, NJ: Erlbaum.

Kazdin, A. E. (1992). *Research design in clinical psychology* (2nd ed.). Boston: Allyn & Bacon.

Kazdin, A. E. (1999). The meanings and measurement of clinical significance. *Journal of Consulting and Clinical Psychology, 67,* 332–339.

Kazdin, A. E. (2000). *Psychotherapy for children and adolescents: Directions for research and practice.* New York: Oxford University Press.

Kendall, P. C., Marrs-Garcia, A., Nath, S. R., & Sheldrick, R. C. (1999). Normative comparisons for the evaluation of clinical significance. *Journal of Consulting and Clinical Psychology, 67,* 285–299.

Klem, L. (2000). Structural equation modeling. In L. G. Grimm & P. R. Yarnold

(Eds.), *Reading and understanding more multivariate statistics* (pp. 227–260). Washington, DC: American Psychological Association.

Knight, G. P., & Hill, N. E. (1998). Measurement equivalence in research involving minority adolescents. In V. C. McLoyd & L. Steinberg (Eds.), *Studying minority adolescents: Conceptual, methodological, and theoretical issues* (pp. 183–210). Mahwah, NJ: Erlbaum.

McConaughy, S. H., & Leone, P. E. (2001). Measuring the success of prevention programs. In B. Algozzine & P. Kay (Eds.), *Preventing problem behaviors: A handbook of successful prevention strategies* (pp. 183–219). Thousand Oaks, CA: Corwin Press.

Muthén, B. (2001). Second-generation structural equation modeling with a combination of categorical and continuous latent variables: New opportunities for latent class-latent growth modeling. In L. M. Collins & A. G. Sayer (Eds.), *New methods for the analysis of change* (pp. 289–322). Washington, DC: American Psychological Association.

Nastasi, B. K., Varjas, K., Schensul, S. L., Silva, K. T., Schensul, J. J., & Ratnayake, P. (2000). The Participatory Intervention Model: A framework for conceptualizing and promoting intervention acceptability. *School Psychology Quarterly, 15*, 207–232.

Nolan, E. E., & Gadow, K. D. (1994). Relation between ratings and observations of stimulant drug response in hyperactive children. *Journal of Clinical Child Psychology, 23*, 78–90.

Pennsylvania Department of Education. (1996). *Every Day, :Lots of Ways: An interdisciplinary nutrition curriculum.* State College, PA: Pennsylvania State Nutrition Department.

Power, T. J., Dowrick, P. W., Ginsburg-Block, M., & Manz, P. H. (2002). *Building the capacity of urban schools to improve literacy skills: Community-assisted tutoring.* Manuscript submitted for publication.

Reid, R., DuPaul, G. J., Power, T. J., Anastopoulos, A. D., Rodgers-Adkinson, D., Noll, M. B., & Riccio, C. (1998). Assessing culturally different students for attention-deficit/hyperactivity disorder using behavior rating scales. *Journal of Abnormal Child Psychology, 26*, 187–198.

Reimers, T. M., Wacker, D. P., Cooper, L. J., & DeRaad, A. O. (1992). Acceptability of behavioral treatments for children: Analog and naturalistic evaluation by parents. *School Psychology Review, 21*, 628–643.

Reimers, T. M., Wacker, D. P., & Koeppl, G. (1987). Acceptability of behavioral interventions: A review of the literature. *School Psychology Review, 16*, 212–227.

Ringwalt, C., Greene, J., Ennett, S., Iachan, R., Clayton, R. R., & Leukefeld, C. G. (1994). Past and future directions of the DARE program: An evaluation review (Award #91–DD-CX-K053). Washington, DC: National Institute of Justice.

Roosa, M. W., Dumka, L. E., Gonzales, N. A., & Knight, G. P. (2002, January 15). Cultural/ethnic issues and the prevention scientist in the 21st century. *Prevention and Treatment, 5*, Article 5. Retrieved October 8, 2001, from *http://journals.apa.org/prevention/volume5/pre0050005a.html*.

Schafer, J. L. (2001). Multiple imputation with PAN. In L. M. Collins & A. G.

Sayer (Eds.), *New methods for the analysis of change* (pp. 355–378). Washington, DC: American Psychological Association.

Sheridan, S. M., & Steck, M. C. (1995). Acceptability of conjoint behavioral consultation: A national survey of school psychologists. *School Psychology Review, 24,* 633–647.

U.S. Department of Health and Human Services. (2000). *2000 dietary guidelines for Americans* (5th ed.). Washington, DC: Author.

Willett, J. B., & Singer, J. D. (1993). Investigating onset, cessation, relapse, and recovery: Why you should, and how you can, use discrete-time survival analysis to examine event occurrence. *Journal of Consulting and Clinical Psychology, 61,* 952–965.

Witt, J. C., & Elliott, S. N. (1985). Acceptability of classroom intervention strategies. In T. R. Kratochwill (Ed.), *Advances in school psychology* (Vol. 4, pp. 251–288). Hillsdale, NJ: Erlbaum.

PART IV

Planning for the Future

CHAPTER 10

Preparing Psychologists to Integrate Systems of Care

As we have described throughout this book, reforms in education and healthcare, as well as advancements in the fields of psychology, education, and medicine, have created the need for professionals who can link systems of care to manage health problems and promote children's healthy development. Historically, training programs in psychology have been designed to educate students to work within particular settings and to focus on discrete domains of child development (La Greca & Hughes, 1999). For example, pediatric psychologists generally have been trained to work in hospital settings and to focus on promoting the healthy development of children with illness and disability. Clinical child psychologists typically have been trained to work in mental healthcare settings and to promote the social and emotional development of children with psychological disorders. Community psychologists are schooled to work in formal and informal community-based systems and to focus on promoting children's mental health. Family psychologists are trained to conduct systemic interventions in a range of settings, although children often are not the direct focus of their work. And school psychologists are prepared to work in educational settings and focus principally on promoting the cognitive and social development of children in school.

In addition, psychology training programs traditionally have endorsed a deficit-oriented model for understanding and addressing the needs of children and their families (Seligman & Csikszentmihalyi, 2000). The emphasis has been on identifying problems and providing services to reduce deficits (Kolbe, Collins, & Cortese, 1997). Training programs have placed much less emphasis on the identification of child and system assets and development of programs to reduce risk and to promote competence.

The preparation of child-oriented psychologists to integrate systems of care and to emphasize competence promotion and risk reduction requires an examination of goals and methods of training. Fortunately, several important reports have been developed that provide guidelines for evaluating training programs and shaping the process of change. The purpose of this chapter is to (1) review recent guidelines for preparing child-oriented psychologists; (2) describe key components of training to prepare child-oriented psychologists to integrate systems of care, with a focus on prevention and intervention; and (3) describe model initiatives situated in university and clinical child psychology training programs.

TRAINING GUIDELINES FOR CHILD-ORIENTED PSYCHOLOGISTS

Over the years, numerous task forces have been created to develop training guidelines for child-oriented psychologists (see La Greca & Hughes, 1999, for a review of developments in training since the 1970s). The following is a brief description of three sets of guidelines developed recently to prepare child-oriented psychologists to respond to reforms in healthcare, mental health, and education.

National Institute of Mental Health Task Group

The National Institute of Mental Health (NIMH) Task Group convened in 1992 to establish guidelines for the preparation of psychologists to serve the needs of children and adolescents. A distinguishing feature was that this task force included clinical child, pediatric, school, community, and family psychologists for the purpose of delineating guidelines for all child-focused psychologists. This task force identified 11 principal areas of training, which are summarized by Roberts et al. (1998; see Table 10.1 for a brief description of each area). These areas have since been used to delineate core areas of training for pediatric psychologists (Spirito et al., in press).

This task force emphasized that students need a solid foundation in principles of developmental psychology, with emphasis on understanding how children develop in multiple systems, including family, school, and peer groups. As outlined in the task force report, training in developmental psychopathology provides a strong basis for designing strategies of intervention and prevention to interrupt pathways to antisocial behavior, emotional disturbance, and poor health outcomes. Comprehensive preparation in assessment includes strategies to evaluate the

TABLE 10.1. Key Training Recommendations of the NIMH Task Group to Refine Clinical Training Guidelines for Services to Children and Adolescents

Domain of training	Description
Developmental psychology	Focuses on the development of individuals across the lifespan within their ecological contexts.
Developmental psychopathology	Focuses on developmental pathways, including an examination of risk and protective factors associated with mental health disorders.
Assessment	Includes methods of assessing the intellectual, personality, and behavioral functioning of children as well as the systems in which children function.
Intervention	Includes interventions for children and the systems in which they develop (family therapy; school, community, and hospital consultation).
Professional, ethical, and legal issues	Focuses on a wide range of professional, ethical, and legal issues that may vary across systems and states.
Research methods and program evaluation	Focuses on research methodology, data analysis, and program evaluation strategies.
Diversity issues and multicultural competence	Focuses on understanding the role of ethnicity and culture in assessing, treating, and preventing health and mental health problems.
Prevention and health promotion	Focuses on program development and evaluation related to programming to prevent risk and to promote healthy development.
Integrating multiple disciplines and systems	Includes strategies for promoting interprofessional, interagency, and family–professional collaboration.
Social issues	Includes a focus on addressing the effects of poverty, discrimination, violence, disasters, and family disruption on children's lives.

Note. Recommendations were derived from the NIMH Task Force group report (see Roberts et al., 1998).

functioning of children, as well as the ecologies in which they develop. Emphasis should be placed on learning culturally sensitive methods of intervention and prevention. The report also recommended that research training is essential to enable students to evaluate research critically and to conduct investigations that promote more effective care for children and their families. Furthermore, the preparation of psychologists ought to include training to work effectively with professionals from multiple disciplines to link systems of care to provide coordinated services to children and their families.

American Psychological Association—Practice Directorate Task Force

A task force was initiated in 1996 by the Practice Directorate of the American Psychological Association (APA) to establish standards for practice and training for professionals in child and adolescent psychology. Like the NIMH task force, this group consisted of professionals from diverse areas of child-oriented psychology. This task force identified several core competencies for the preparation of psychologists serving the needs of children and adolescents (American Psychological Association, 1998); these are summarized in Table 10.2.

This APA task force stressed the importance of preparing professionals to understand that development is strongly influenced by an individual's culture and context, and that differentiating normal from pathological pathways of development requires an understanding of the family in the context of the culture in which it functions. Effective practice requires the application of empirically supported strategies and responsiveness to culturally determined beliefs about the goals and methods of intervention. This task force highlighted the importance of acquiring skills in intersystemic collaboration to promote the coordination of care for children and families. In addition, the need for professional training in skills of program development (e.g., team building and grant writing), implementation (e.g., recruitment and training of professional and paraprofessional staff, manualization of treatment, and integrity monitoring), and evaluation (e.g., scale development, between- and within-

TABLE 10.2. Core Competencies for Doctoral and Internship Training outlined by the APA Task Force on Child and Adolescent Professional Psychology

---

Culturally responsive assessment and intervention services

Collaborative and interprofessional relationships

Brief, empirically supported interventions

Focused assessment methods that are directly linked to problem solving

Program evaluation and outcome assessment

Program and professional development skills, including grant writing and marketing

Administration, supervisory, and staff development skills

Note. Core competencies were derived from the Report of the APA Task Force on Child and Adolescent Professional Psychology (American Psychological Association, 1998).

group designs, and single-subject design) was highlighted (La Greca & Hughes, 1999).

National Association of School Psychologists—Blueprint

The National Association of School Psychologists (NASP) convened a task force in the mid-1990s to develop core domains of practice and training for school psychologists (Ysseldyke et al., 1997). The report issued by this committee, *School Psychology: A Blueprint for Training and Practice II*, identified 10 core domains, which are listed and described briefly in Table 10.3.

Many of the domains identified in the NASP blueprint overlap with core areas specified by the NIMH and APA task forces. Specifically, all three groups stressed the importance of developing skills related to (1) assessing individual children, as well as the systems in which they function; (2) designing strategies of prevention, as well as intervention; (3) promoting partnerships across systems of care; (4) providing services in a culturally sensitive manner; (5) linking research with practice and evaluating outcomes; and (6) understanding ethical and legal standards related to practice and research. The NASP guidelines are unique in that they emphasize the importance of understanding school ecology and creating interventions to promote the development of cognitive and academic skills. Although the NASP blueprint was developed to set standards for school psychology practice, its guidelines are useful in identifying core domains of competence for child-oriented psychologists whose professional activities include a focus on intervention and prevention (see Power, 2002).

TABLE 10.3. Domains of School Psychology Training and Practice

Data-based decision making and accountability
Interpersonal communication, collaboration, and consultation
Effective instruction and development of cognitive/academic skills
Socialization and development of life competencies
Student diversity in development and learning
School structure, organization, and climate
Prevention, wellness promotion, and crisis intervention
Home–school–community collaboration
Research and program evaluation
Legal, ethical practice, and professional development

Note. Domains were derived from Ysseldyke et al. (1997).

CORE DOMAINS OF TRAINING

The guidelines developed by NIMH, APA, and NASP provide a strong foundation for delineating core domains for the preparation of child-focused psychologists to respond creatively to the challenges of health-care, mental healthcare, and education reform. Core domains addressed by each of these task forces include developmental–ecological psychology, developmental psychopathology, multimodal assessment, empirically supported and socially valid intervention, prevention and health promotion, multicultural competence, multisystemic collaboration, theory and practice of organizational change, research methods, program development and evaluation, professional issues, and learning experiences in multiple settings. The following is a description of these core components.

Developmental–Ecological Psychology

Practice and research in child-oriented psychology must be firmly rooted in developmental psychology across the lifespan. Psychologists need to understand how children, adolescents, and adults develop in the context of the major ecologies in which they function (Bronfenbrenner, 1979). Individuals create and are shaped by the contexts in which they develop. The quality of relationships in each of the major systems of a child's life, such as parent–child, teacher–child, and peer–child systems, is critical for positive, healthy development (Pianta, 1997). The ability of a child to function in a system is highly influenced by relationships between members of that system and individuals from other systems. Furthermore, the preparation requires that child-oriented psychologists understand how cultural factors influence the development of children by impacting on family, school, and healthcare systems and the relationships among them.

Developmental Psychopathology

Research related to developmental psychopathology forms an important foundation for the science and practice of prevention. Child-oriented psychologists need to understand developmental pathways leading to psychopathology and poor health outcomes. For example, researchers have identified developmental pathways associated with the emergence of anxiety disorders (Donovan & Spence, 2000), depressive disorders (Cicchetti & Toth, 1998), and antisocial behavior disorders (Loeber & Stouthamer-Loeber, 1998; Patterson, Reid, & Dishion, 1992). This research has been highly successful in identifying variables associated with risk for psychopathology, as well as factors that promote effective coping and resilience (Masten & Coatsworth, 1998). Effective prevention programs are firmly based in research in developmental psychopathology. These programs target children known to be at heightened risk for mental and physical health problems, and include multiple intervention components designed to reduce risk and build resilience.

Multimodal Assessment

Training needs to emphasize that assessment is relevant only to the extent that it leads to the design of effective, useful, and socially valid strategies to resolve problems and/or promote competence (Roberts et al., 1998). Comprehensive training necessitates preparation in methods of assessing a broad range of function, including cognitive, academic, social, emotional, and behavioral domains. Several modes of assessment are useful in creating strategies designed to change individual children and the contexts in which they function, and to improve important relationships in their lives (see Chapter 3). These methods include (1) developmental and behavioral assessment to determine the child's cognitive, academic, social, emotional, and behavioral functioning in relationship to children of similar age and gender; (2) diagnostic assessment to evaluate the presence of psychopathology or risk for disturbance; (3) ecological assessment to determine factors in the child's ecologies that promote and serve as barriers to development; and (4) functional assessment to identify potential relationships among environmental conditions (e.g., reinforcement contingencies) and the child's behavior. Child-oriented psychologists need to understand the strengths and limitations of each method, and how these approaches may complement one another and be combined in practice (see Chapter 3).

Empirically Supported and Socially Valid Intervention

Child-oriented psychologists need to know how to evaluate the research literature critically to determine whether an intervention strategy is efficacious. Knowledge about the status of research related to the treatment of various pediatric conditions and child mental health disorders is important. At the same time, an understanding of the difference between efficacious and effective intervention, and the challenges of developing effective programs in diverse settings is essential (Dodge, 2001; see Chapter 11). A critical concept related to intervention is social validity, that is, the extent to which the goals, methods, and outcomes of intervention are viewed as reasonable, fair, and appropriate by participants or stakeholders (Schwartz & Baer, 1991). Developing potentially effective interventions is a dialectical process that occurs in the context of an ongoing partnership between the intervention specialist and participants, and seeks to achieve a balance between guidelines based on empirical research and participant beliefs about what is acceptable and valuable (Fantuzzo & Mohr, 2000).

Prevention and Health Promotion

Responding to the challenges of reform requires that child-oriented psychologists be prepared in the areas of prevention and health promotion, including the three levels of prevention: universal, selective, and indicated (see Chapters 7 and 8). Child-oriented psychologists need to understand how research in developmental psychology and psychopathology serves as the basis for the science and practice of prevention. Furthermore, training in the principles of effective prevention programming is essential. Effective programs of prevention have a dual goal of reducing health risk and promoting competence (Masten & Coatsworth, 1998). These programs focus on changing individual children by improving skills; altering the contexts in which children develop by changing the family, school, and healthcare systems; and improving relationships in the family, school, community, and peer systems (Pianta & Walsh, 1998). Successful programs are developed in partnership with all participants who have a stake in the program.

Multicultural Competence

A focus on diversity issues and multicultural competence ought to permeate all components of training. The development of children is strongly influenced by the culture of the family and community in which they function. Discontinuities between the cultures of different systems in which children develop can serve as a significant barrier to the promotion of competence in children (Comer, Haynes, Joyner, & Ben-Avie, 1996). Determinations about whether a behavior is a problem, whether a problem is viewed as requiring intervention, and who is the most appropriate service provider are influenced greatly by cultural factors (Sue & Sue, 1999). Assessment, intervention, and prevention strategies need to be developed in a manner that is responsive to the culturally determined beliefs and values of the families being served. In addition, research ought to be developed in partnership with participants from the various cultures represented to ensure its meaningfulness and social validity (Nastasi et al., 2000; see Chapter 11).

Multisystemic Collaboration

Child-focused psychologists need to be trained in strategies of collaborative consultation with professionals from a wide range of disciplines pertaining to healthcare, mental healthcare, and education. Furthermore, instruction is required in methods of promoting intersystem partnerships to address the health needs of children and their families. The Conjoint Behavioral Consultation Model (Sheridan, Kratochwill, & Bergan, 1996; see Chapter 4), which integrates systems and behavioral perspectives to promote collaborative problem solving between families and schools, is highly useful in preparing child-oriented psychologists for collaborative practice. This model can be adapted to include the health system, along with the family and school systems, in the process of collaboration (see Chapter 3). Also, reframing the focus of the model to include competence promotion, in addition to problem solving, is consistent with recent contributions from intervention and prevention researchers (Cicchetti & Toth, 1998; Pianta & Walsh, 1998).

Theory and Practice of Organizational Change

Being a child-oriented psychologist involves the ability to work effectively in multiple systems and to facilitate effective partnerships across systems (Knoff, 1996). School psychologists generally receive considerable training with regard to the ecology of schools and strategies for working effectively in this system. Unfortunately, their training related to the healthcare and mental healthcare systems may be limited. Similarly, pediatric and clinical child psychologists generally are better trained to work in healthcare and mental healthcare systems, but they typically have limited training in school systems (Power, DuPaul, Shapiro, & Parrish, 1995). Even when child-oriented psychologists are prepared to work in a specific system, their training may be focused primarily on strategies to change individual children. They may not be prepared to change the ecology, so that it better serves the needs of children and is linked effectively with other major systems in the child's life.

Research Methods

Instruction in research methods needs to be initiated at the beginning of training and should continue throughout its course. Child-oriented psychologists need to know how to evaluate research critically and translate research findings into implications for practice and future research (see Chapter 11). In addition, it is important for child-oriented psychologists to have the skills needed to contribute to theory development and practice by conducting their own original research. Research training includes a focus on methods of developing and validating assessment measures, prediction strategies using regression methods, group design methods for evaluating outcome, and single-subject outcome strategies (Roberts et al., 1998). Opportunities for developing advanced skills in research methods can be provided for individuals who wish to pursue careers primarily devoted to research.

Program Development and Evaluation

Child-oriented psychologists generally receive little training related to the development and evaluation of programs in community settings in part nership with diverse stakeholder groups. In response to reforms, child-oriented psychology is shifting to include a public health perspective, which focuses on creating health promotion programs for a large group of children, in addition to a service delivery approach, which focuses on problem solving for an individual child (Power, 2000; Short & Talley, 1997). Child-focused psychologists can benefit from training in methods of developing and evaluating programs that can have an impact at a systemic level and effect the outcomes of many children and families. Methods of participatory action research are highly useful in developing programs that are responsive to the needs of multiple stakeholder groups in the community (Nastasi et al., 2000; see Chapter 7). Training in grant writing is critical to secure funding from public and private sources to develop and validate these initiatives (American Psychological Association, 1998).

Professional, Ethical, and Legal Issues

A wide range of ethical and legal issues must be addressed in child-oriented psychology training programs (Koocher & Keith-Spiegel, 1998). A critical concern that arises in work that spans multiple systems of care is the difference in ethical and legal standards of practice that apply in healthcare versus mental healthcare versus educational settings. Child-focused psychologists ought to conduct their clinical and research activities in a manner that is consistent with legal and professional guidelines for practice that may vary across systems, while adhering to the ethical code outlined by the APA. For example, providing healthcare and mental healthcare services in schools can be challenging because of differences in standards of practice for protecting privacy within these settings. Also, the increasing use of computer technology raises challenging concerns to psychologists relative to the protection of privacy in maintaining electronic records and communicating with professionals via the Internet (Kruger, 2001).

Learning Experiences in Multiple Settings

Because child-oriented psychologists require instruction related to health-care, mental healthcare, and education, their training may need to span two or more university-based academic schools or departments, such as schools of arts and science, education, and medicine (Power, Shapiro, & DuPaul, in press; Roberts, 1998). Exposure to an interdisciplinary faculty during graduate school may help students to acquire the breadth of training needed and to learn strategies for collaborating with professionals from a wide range of disciplines. Practicum experiences should be offered in a wide range of settings, including primary and tertiary healthcare settings, mental healthcare settings, and schools (Power, Manz, & Leff, in press). Field supervisors may include child clinical, pediatric, school, family, and community psychologists. Professionals in other disciplines, such as child psychiatrists, pediatricians, nurses, public health specialists, social workers, and guidance counselors, may provide mentoring and supplemental supervision.

MODEL DOCTORAL TRAINING PROGRAMS

Many pathways are available for the preparation of child-oriented psychologists to integrate systems of care, with a focus on managing and preventing health problems. Although numerous child-oriented doctoral training programs have been adapted to respond to the challenges of healthcare and educational reform, we highlight two programs that have served as models for training in school psychology and clinical child psychology.

Training Nested in a School Psychology Program

In 1997, through the collaborative efforts of Lehigh University and the Children's Hospital of Philadelphia (CHOP), a program linking pediatric and school psychology was established (Shapiro, DuPaul, & Power, 1997). This program, which was initially funded in 1997 by the U.S. Department of Education, Office of Special Education, and was refunded in 2001, is nested in the APA-approved School Psychology Training Program within the College of Education at Lehigh University. The program reflects a partnership between faculty in the Colleges of Education and Arts and Sciences at Lehigh, and faculty at CHOP, which serves at the Department of Pediatrics for the University of Pennsylvania School of Medicine. Students may elect to enroll in this program in the third and fourth years of their doctoral studies.

Program Goals

The goal of the Lehigh–CHOP program is to prepare scientist–practitioners to link the family, school, healthcare, and mental healthcare systems of care to manage and prevent children's chronic health conditions, including mental health disorders. The program has a dual focus on preparing professionals in the domains of service delivery and public health. In the domain of service delivery, students are trained to address the needs of one or more children who have identified health conditions or are at-risk for health problems because of emotional and behavioral difficulties. In the domain of public health, students are trained to develop and evaluate programs for large groups of children to prevent health risk and to promote healthy development (Power, Shapiro, & DuPaul, in press). The Lehigh–CHOP initiative is especially designed to prepare child-oriented psychologists to address the needs of children and families from highly diverse cultural backgrounds that reside in underserved, urban neighborhoods. Students in this program are expected to attain competencies in four domains, in addition to the four domains of training that have been established for all students in the School Psychology Program (see Table 10.4 for a description of each set of training domains).

Coursework

In the first 2 years of doctoral study, trainees are required to take core courses in psychology (e.g., social and developmental bases of human behavior), as well courses in the historical roots of school psychology, assessment, intervention, and assessment. Courses specific to the Lehigh–CHOP initiative are taken in the third and fourth years of study (see Table 10.5 for a list of courses taken by most students). The core courses in this specialization program comprise a yearlong seminar related to strategies of intervention for children with, or at risk for, health problems, taken in the third year, and a yearlong seminar related to prevention and health promotion, taken in the fourth year. The seminar in prevention provides advanced training in program development and evaluation, as well as grant writing. Additional courses taken in the third and fourth years include courses in child psychopathology, neuropharmacology, organizational management, child and family intervention, multicultural counseling, and an advanced seminar in child development.

Courses are taken in a university (Lehigh) and a medical school (CHOP) setting. Professors at Lehigh include faculty in the College of Arts and Sciences, including the Psychology and Biology Departments, as well as faculty in the College of Education, including the Psychology, Counseling Psychology, Special Education, and Educational Leadership

TABLE 10.4. Competency Domains for the Standard Doctoral Program at Lehigh University and Additional Domains for the Lehigh–CHOP Specialization Program

Competency domain	Description
	Standard Lehigh doctoral program
1. Core psychological knowledge	Knowledge of the biological and social bases of behavior. Knowledge of how children develop in the context of multiple systems.
2. Research design and application	Knowledge and application of single-subject, group, and correlational research designs.
3. Psychological applications	Knowledge and application of assessment and intervention methods to address academic, social, emotional, and behavioral problems.
4. Professional/multicultural issues	Knowledge and application of ethical principles in providing services and conducting research; application of services to children and families from diverse cultural backgrounds.
	Lehigh–CHOP specialization program
5. Interventions for chronic illness	Knowledge of medical conditions and application of interventions to address the needs of children coping with chronic illness.
6. Prevention programming	Knowledge and application of principles of developmental psychopathology and positive psychology to design prevention programs.
7. Program evaluation	Use of single-subject, quasi-experimental, and participatory action research methods to evaluate program outcomes.
8. Intersystem collaboration	Expertise in addressing health problems in multiple settings and in linking systems to provide coordinated services for children and families.

programs. Two of the courses offered at CHOP are taught by faculty in the Department of Psychology and Division of Developmental and Behavioral Pediatrics of CHOP, many of whom hold appointments in the University of Pennsylvania School of Medicine.

Practicum Experiences

A hallmark of the Lehigh–CHOP initiative is the integrated set of practicum experiences in medical and school settings. During the third

TABLE 10.5. Sample Listing of Coursework for Students Enrolled in the Lehigh–CHOP Training Program

First year—fall semester
   Social Basis of Human Behavior (3)
   Historical and Contemporary Issues in School Psychology (3)
   Applied Behavior Analysis (3)
   Applied Research Practicum (1)
First year—spring semester
   Developmental Psychology (3)
   Assessment of Intelligence (3)
   Single-Case Research Design (3)
   Practicum in the Assessment of Intelligence (1)
First year—summer
   Multicultural Issues (3)
Second year—fall semester
   Univariate Statistical Models (3)
   Behavioral Assessment (3)
   Consultation Procedures (2)
   Practicum in Consultation (1)
   Practicum in Behavioral Assessment (1)
Second year—spring semester
   Assessment and Intervention in Educational Consultation (3)
   Advanced School and Family Interventions (3)
   Multivariate Statistical Models (3)
   Practicum in Assessment and Intervention in Educational Consultation (1)
Second year—summer
   Behavioral Neuroscience (3)
Third year—fall semester
   Health/Pediatric Psychology (3)
   Theory and Practice of Organizational Development (3)
   Doctoral Qualifying Project (3)
   Doctoral Practicum in Pediatric School Psychology (1)
Third year—spring semester
   Application in Pediatric School Psychology—Intervention (3)
   Advanced Child Psychopathology (3)
   Special Education elective (3)
   Doctoral Practicum in Pediatric School Psychology (1)
Third year—summer
   Neuropharmacology (3)
Fourth year—fall semester
   Comprehensive School Health Programs (3)
   Advanced Applications in Psychometrics (3)
   Counseling Psychology elective (3)
   Doctoral Practicum in Pediatric School Psychology (1)
Fourth year—spring semester
   Applications in Pediatric School Psychology—Prevention (3)
   Advanced Seminar in Child Development (3)
   Advanced Research Methods (3)
   Doctoral Practicum in Pediatric School Psychology (1)
Fifth year—full year
   Internship

Note. Credit hours for each course are indicated in parentheses.

and fourth years of study, students are placed in both types of settings (see Shapiro, DuPaul, Power, Gureasko, & Moore, 2000). Healthcare practica are offered in primary and secondary care settings in the Lehigh Valley, as well as in a tertiary care setting (CHOP). At CHOP, students are placed in the Center for Management of ADHD and the Behavioral Pediatrics, Gastroenterology, Neonatal Follow-Up, Pain Management, Adherence, and Oncology programs. In their healthcare practica, students are supervised by faculty from Lehigh and CHOP, as well as other licensed psychologists and pediatricians, including specialists in Developmental and Behavior Pediatrics.

School practica are served in the Allentown School District and the School District of Philadelphia. Both districts serve children from highly diverse ethnic and cultural backgrounds. During these experiences, trainees have the opportunity to develop skills related to typical school psychology practice, including assessment and consultation skills. In addition, students are expected to provide services to children with chronic illnesses, including mental health disorders, and to develop and evaluate prevention and health promotion programs. School practica are supervised by faculty from Lehigh and CHOP, in addition to school psychologists based at the sites.

Research Training

During the 2-year specialization program, students are encouraged to conduct research related to children's health issues, which can include investigations designed to understand the challenges that children with health problems encounter in schools, families, and community systems, as well as research focused on identifying, managing, and preventing health issues. Examples include developing and evaluating school-based asthma prevention and nutrition education programs, and developing health promotion programs in primary care settings. Course assignments are designed to assist students in conducting their research. For example, students are expected to prepare literature reviews, journal article critiques, a grant proposal, and an institutional review board (IRB) proposal related to their research conducted for qualifying projects and dissertations. Furthermore, in their practicum placement, trainees are encouraged to select cases and develop programs of intervention or prevention related to proposed topics for their dissertation. In addition, students have multiple opportunities to collaborate on projects headed by the faculty. Many students are involved as coauthors of national presentations (e.g., Manz, Power, Coniglio, & Gureasko, 2000; Moore & DuPaul, 2001), journal articles (e.g., Hoffman & DuPaul, 2000), newsletter articles (e.g., Shapiro et al., 2000), and book chapters (e.g., DuPaul, McGoey, & Mautone, in press) during the course of their doctoral studies.

Training Nested in a Clinical Child/Pediatric Psychology Program

In 1991, through the collaborative efforts of the Clinical Psychology Program of the Department of Psychology and the Human Development and Family Life Department of the College of Liberal Arts and Sciences of the University of Kansas (KU), the Clinical Child Psychology Program (CCPP) was established (Roberts, 1998). Close collaboration with university-affiliated hospitals, and local school districts and mental health agencies, has been critical to the success of the program. CCPP has two tracks: (1) clinical psychology focused on providing a broad range of mental health services to children and adolescents, and (2) pediatric psychology.

Program Goals

The training recommendations developed by the NIMH-sponsored task group (Roberts et al., 1998), which are summarized in Table 10.1, serve as the foundation for CCPP. From its outset, CCPP was designed to be an innovative, interdepartmental program integrating principles and perspectives from developmental, ecological, and clinical psychology in the preparation of scientist–practitioners. This program strives to prepare students to (1) understand development in the context of the major systems in which children develop; (2) understand developmental pathways leading to pathology, as well as risk and protective factors that influence the course of development; (3) provide intervention and prevention services in a manner that is consistent with empirically supported practice and responsive to the culture and ethnicity of children and their families; (4) promote interdisciplinary collaboration and partnerships among individuals from multiple systems; and (5) consider ethical and legal issues related to research and practice with children and adolescents in diverse settings (Roberts, 1998).

Coursework

Required coursework includes foundational courses in psychology, as well as specialty courses in clinical child psychology. For students who choose the pediatric psychology track, several optional courses in pediatric psychology are available. (See Roberts & Steele, in press, for a list of core courses and electives in pediatric psychology.) The courses in pediatric psychology provide training in the physiological and psychological aspects of health and disease, developmental disabilities, and specialty topics such as treatment adherence (Roberts & Steele, in press).

Courses have been designed so that they address the breadth of recommendations outlined by the NIMH task force on clinical training related to services for children and adolescents. Courses are taught by core faculty within CCPP, as well as other faculty members from the Departments of Psychology and Human Development and Family Life, and faculty from affiliated institutions, such as the KU Medical Center and Children's Mercy Hospital (Roberts & Steele, in press).

Practicum Experiences

Providing practicum training in a manner that is highly integrated with coursework and that addresses the NIMH task force recommendations is a hallmark of CCPP (Roberts, 1998). Early in their doctoral studies, students in CCPP receive training in the KU Child and Family Services Clinic under the supervision of CCPP faculty members, as well as adjunct-faculty clinicians from the community. Subsequently, students in the pediatric track may elect the following rotations: Child Development Unit at KU Medical Center, in which students receive training in interdisciplinary evaluation for children with chronic illnesses and disabilities; Children's Mercy Hospital, in which trainees have the opportunity to provide therapy and consultation/liaison services in outpatient and inpatient settings; and the Pediatric Psychology Unit at KU Medical Center, through which students can elect rotations in outpatient therapy for children with disruptive disorders, consultation and therapy in a primary care pediatric clinic, and consultation/liaison on inpatient medical units.

Students also have opportunities to receive training in community mental healthcare settings and schools. Of particular note, the Elementary Therapeutic Classroom (ECT), a collaborative effort of KU and a local school district, provides comprehensive mental healthcare services in schools to children with emotional, behavioral, and learning problems, who have problems coping in the classroom. Through the ECT, students receive training in interdisciplinary collaboration in school settings to address the needs of children with or at risk for chronic illnesses, serious behavioral or emotional problems, and developmental disabilities (Roberts & Steele, in press).

Research Training

Advanced training in research methods is a critical component of CCPP. In addition to the dissertation project, students have opportunities to collaborate with faculty on numerous research teams during the course of the program (Roberts & Steele, in press). Students gain experience with a broad range of content areas and methodologies, including (1) the development of measures for assessing adherence, coping with illness, and addressing vocational aspirations of children with chronic illness; (2) outcome evaluation of treatments to improve adherence to medical regimens for numerous chronic illnesses; and (3) program evaluation of outpatient services and camps designed for children with chronic illness. A high percentage of students in CCPP serve as coauthors of journal manuscripts, book chapters, and presentations at national conferences. Faculty often request students to assist with the review of journal articles submitted for publication. In addition, students have the opportunity to gain experience with grant writing and other grant preparation activities.

INTERNSHIP AND FELLOWSHIP TRAINING

We propose that training at the internship and fellowship levels provide an integrated set of applied, mentored experiences related to each of the core domains of training outlined here. The internship and fellowship should offer trainees opportunities to work in multiple systems with professionals from various disciplines, and to contribute to the development and evaluation of intervention and prevention programs for children and families from diverse cultural backgrounds.

Predoctoral Internship Training

During the internship, trainees should have opportunities to engage in a wide range of clinical activities, including assessment, intervention, consultation, prevention, and health promotion with children of varying developmental levels and cultural backgrounds. For example, the Internship Training Program at CHOP, which is accredited by the APA, provides training experiences across a broad range of programs related to clinical child, pediatric, community, and school psychology. Examples of clinical child rotations include the Center for Management of ADHD, the Developmental Assessment Program, the Developmental Neuropsychology Service, and the Child and Family Therapy Service. Pediatric psychology rotations include programs in the Division of Oncology, the Consultation and Liaison Program, the Thoracic Organ Transplant Program, the Pain Management Program, and the Adherence Program. Community and school psychology rotations include Reading Partners, a literacy development initiative based in the schools; the Playground, Lunchroom, and Youth Success program, a school-based violence prevention project; and Project Teach, a community-based initiative to build community partnerships to strengthen out-of-school health promotion programs for youth. Being situated in the Philadelphia metropolitan area, CHOP offers trainees opportunities to address the needs of children from diverse ethnic, cultural, and socioeconomic backgrounds.

The Internship Training Program at CHOP is nested within a Leadership Education in Neurodevelopmental and Related Disabilities (LEND) program funded by the Maternal and Child Health Bureau of the U.S. Department of Health and Human Services, an interdisciplinary program providing education to trainees from 11 disciplines. The LEND program provides interns with ongoing opportunities to learn about the challenges of designing, implementing, and evaluating programs for children and families across multiple systems in an interdisciplinary educational forum.

Although the internship at CHOP is designed principally to provide mentored, clinical experience, interns are given protected time to devote to a research activity. Examples include participation in research related to the Surviving Cancer Competently Intervention Program (SCCIP; see Kazak et al., 1999), a cognitive-behavioral and family therapy intervention program for adolescent survivors of cancer and their families; and the Family–School Success Program (see Power, Russell, Soffer, Blom-Hoffman, & Grim, 2002), a family–school intervention for children with ADHD, which integrates behavioral and family/systems methods.

Most internships are 1 year in duration, which may not provide students with sufficient experience across a broad range of settings to become expert in multisystemic intervention and prevention. Also, the internship typically focuses on clinical training and may be limited with regard to its emphasis on research training. The opportunity to combine the internship year with a year of postdoctoral training may be better suited to the preparation of child-oriented psychologists, particularly those who wish to pursue an academic career. Indeed, at CHOP, interns who have been granted a postdoctoral fellowship have been able to pursue research related to school-based nutrition education, cognitive remediation for adolescents treated for brain tumors, behavioral intervention for children with traumatic brain injury, and sleep intervention for children with chronic illnesses.

Postdoctoral Fellowship Training

Training at the postdoctoral fellowship level can provide opportunities to receive training in settings and domains not sufficiently addressed in the doctoral and/or internship programs. Because the fellowship experience typically affords concentrated training in self-selected areas of interest, opportunities for advanced training related to specific domains of intervention and prevention may be available at this level of preparation.

In addition, the fellowship can afford trainees the academic mentoring they need to launch careers as leaders in program development, teaching, and research. For example, trainees at CHOP have successfully used the fellowship experience to prepare for careers as community-based prevention researchers in the areas of violence prevention and nutrition education. Other fellows have pursued academic careers, with a focus on intervention research related to coping with illness in family, school, and peer systems.

Critical to the success of a fellowship is that the trainee become aligned with one or more mentors who embrace the scientist–practitioner model and are highly invested in the career development of fellows. Because the fellowship program typically is a highly individualized training experience designed collaboratively by the fellow and his or her mentors, it is essential that the fellow work closely with mentors who are committed to helping trainees build successful careers as multisystem change agents. One year of a fellowship often may not be sufficient to launch a career as a leader in linking systems to manage and prevent health problems. In many settings, the option for a second year is available and may provide the additional mentoring needed for the fellow to become a successful leader.

POTENTIAL CHALLENGES

Although the benefits of following the guidelines outlined by the NIMH, APA, and NASP task forces for the preparation of child-oriented psychologist are numerous, a number of challenges can arise in developing and implementing innovative training programs based on these recommendations. As an example, program faculty may have limited preparation in one or more of the core domains addressed by the training guidelines, which may restrict their ability to serve as effective role models and mentors for their students. One way in which this problem was addressed in the Lehigh–CHOP program was to forge partnerships across a university-based training program and a medical school-based program, and to include faculty representing various departments and disciplines. Likewise, the training program at KU incorporates the expertise of faculty across two departments of the university.

Training related to intervention and prevention across multiple systems may require that students spend additional time in their preparation to be psychologists. For example, although the Lehigh–CHOP program does not require additional coursework compared to the standard doctoral-level training program at Lehigh, students are required to have additional practicum experiences (Power, Shapiro, & DuPaul, in press), which may add to the length and cost of training for students. This may be problematic in programs that have limited support for students through extra- and intramural sources.

Another challenge is that health reimbursement systems, largely shaped by the managed care movement, may not support many of the activities that experts in child-oriented psychology have outlined as best practices for our profession. For example, managed care often "carves out" mental health services, which imposes a false dichotomy between healthcare and mental healthcare. To gain access to mental health benefits, it is usually necessary to demonstrate the presence of significant psychiatric deficits or disorders (Roberts & Hurley, 1997). Such a system does not account for and reimburse prevention activities designed to prevent or reduce the impact of health and mental health problems. Furthermore, managed care often does not support interdisciplinary care for illness and mental health problems. Providing training opportunities related to intervention, as well as prevention, and offering students experiences in interdisciplinary contexts often require grant funding from public and private agencies.

CONCLUSIONS

Advancements in public policy and research related to healthcare, mental healthcare, and education have affirmed the need for leaders who can successfully collaborate with professionals from various disciplines in multiple settings and integrate systems of care to manage and prevent health problems. Responding to the challenges of reform has highlighted the need to integrate child-oriented specialties in psychology (e.g., pediatric, clinical child, school, family, and community). For example, pediatric psychologists face the challenge of addressing the health needs of children as they arise in hospital, school, and community settings, and it is important that they coordinate care across these systems. Similarly, school psychologists should be competent in addressing the educational, mental healthcare, and healthcare needs of students in school and community settings.

Recently, leaders in child-oriented psychology have identified a common set of core competencies that need be mastered across training programs nested within various specialties of child-oriented psychology. Task forces within APA and NIMH, consisting of representatives from the various divisions of child-oriented psychology, have endorsed a unified set of guidelines to serve as a framework for training.

Based upon the reports of training task forces sponsored by APA and NIMH, as well as a leadership group within school psychology, this chapter has identified and described core domains of competence for the preparation of child-oriented psychologists to serve as leaders in the linking of systems to develop and evaluate programs of intervention and prevention. Multiple pathways for preparing psychologists to meet the challenges of reform are available. In this chapter, we have presented two potential pathways for training: one nested within a school psychology training program, and the other nested in a clinical child/pediatric psychology program. We propose that predoctoral internship and postdoctoral training programs focus their efforts on providing advanced training related to the core domains of competence outlined in the APA and NIMH task force reports.

REFERENCES

American Psychological Association. (1998). *Report of the Task Force on Child and Adolescent Professional Psychology to the Board of Professional Affairs.* Washington, DC: Author.

Bronfenbrenner, U. (1979). *The ecology of human development.* Cambridge, MA: Harvard University Press.

Cicchetti, D., & Toth, S. L. (1998). The development of depression in children and adolescents. *American Psychologist, 53,* 221–241.

Comer, J. P., Haynes, N. M., Joyner, E. T., & Ben-Avie, M. (1996). *Rallying the whole village: The Comer process for reforming education.* New York: Teachers College Press.

Dodge, K. A. (2001). The science of youth violence prevention: Progressing from developmental epidemiology to efficacy to effectiveness to public policy. *American Journal of Preventive Medicine, 20,* 63–70.

Donovan, C. L., & Spence, S. H. (2000). Prevention of childhood anxiety disorders. *Clinical Psychology Review, 20,* 509–531.

DuPaul, G. J., McGoey, K., & Mautone, J. (in press). Pediatric pharmacology and psychopharmacology. In M. C. Roberts (Ed.), *Handbook of pediatric psychology* (3rd ed.). New York: Guilford Press.

Fantuzzo, J. W., & Mohr, W. (2000). Pursuit of wellness in Head Start: Making beneficial connections for children and families. In D. Cicchetti, J. Rapapport, I. Sandler, & R. Weissberg (Eds.), *The promotion of wellness in children and adolescents* (pp. 463–514). Thousand Oaks, CA: Sage.

Hoffman, J. A., & DuPaul, G. J. (2000). Psychoeducational interventions for attention-deficit/hyperactivity disorder. *Child and Adolescent Psychiatric Clinics of North America, 9,* 647–661.

Kazak, A. Simms, S., Barakat, L., Hobbie, W., Foley, B., Golomb, B., & Best, M. (1999). Surviving Cancer Competently Intervention Program (SCCIP): A cognitive-behavioral and family therapy intervention for adolescent survivors of childhood cancer and their families. *Family Process, 38,* 175–192.

Knoff, H. W. (1996). The interface of school, community, and health care reform:

Organizational directions toward effective services for children and youth. *School Psychology Review, 25,* 446–464.

Kolbe, L. J., Collins, J., & Cortese, P. (1997). Building the capacity of schools to improve the health of the nation: A call for assistance from psychologists. *American Psychologist, 52,* 256–265.

Koocher, G. P., & Keith-Spiegel, P. (1998). *Ethics in psychology: Professional standards and cases* (2nd ed.). New York: Oxford University Press.

Kruger, L. J. (Ed.). (2001). *Computers in the delivery of special education and related services: Developing collaborative and individualized learning environments.* Binghamton, NY: Haworth Press.

La Greca, A. M., & Hughes, J. N. (1999). United we stand, divided we fall: The education and training of clinical child psychologists. *Journal of Clinical Child Psychology, 28,* 435–447.

Loeber, R., & Stouthamer-Loeber, M. (1998). Development of juvenile aggression and violence: Some common misconceptions and controversies. *American Psychologist, 53,* 242–259.

Manz, P. H., Power, T. J., Coniglio, J., & Gureasko, S. (2000, March). *Celebrating our communities' success: Lessons in establishing effective community partnership interventions in urban schools.* Workshop presented at the annual conference of the National Association of School Psychologists, New Orleans, LA.

Masten, A. S., & Coatsworth, J. D. (1998). The development of competence in favorable and unfavorable environments: Lessons from research on successful children. *American Psychologist, 53,* 205–220.

Moore, D., & DuPaul, G. J. (2001, April). *Expanding school psychologists' roles: Increasing adherence to asthma medication regimens.* Poster presented at the annual conference of the National Association of School Psychologists, Washington, DC.

Nastasi, B. K., Varjas, K., Schensul, S. L., Silva, K. T., Schensul, J. J., & Ratnayake, P. (2000). The participatory intervention model: A framework for conceptualizing and promoting intervention acceptability. *School Psychology Quarterly, 15,* 207–232.

Patterson, G., Reid, J., & Dishion, T. (1992). *Antisocial boys.* Eugene, OR: Castalia.

Pianta, R. C. (1997). Adult–child relationship processes and early schooling. *Early Education and Development, 8,* 11–26.

Pianta, R. C., & Walsh, D. J. (1998). Applying the construct of resilience in schools: Cautions from a developmental systems perspective. *School Psychology Review, 27,* 407–417.

Power, T. J. (2000). Commentary: The school psychologist as community-focused, public health professional: Emerging challenges and implications for training. *School Psychology Review, 29,* 557–559.

Power, T. J. (2002). Preparing school psychologists as interventionists and preventionists. In M. R. Shinn, H. M. Walker, & G. Stoner (Eds.), *Interventions for academic and behavior problems: II. Preventive and remedial approaches* (pp. 1047–1065). Bethesda, MD: National Association of School Psychologists.

Power, T. J., DuPaul, G. J., Shapiro, E. S., & Parrish, J. M. (1995). Pediatric school psychology: The emergence of a subspecialty. *School Psychology Review, 24,* 244–257.

Power, T. J., Manz, P. H., & Leff, S. S. (in press). Training for effective practice in schools. In M. Weist, S. Evans, & N. Tashman (Eds.), *School mental health handbook.* Norwell, MA: Kluwer Academic/Plenum Press.

Power, T. J., Russell, H. F., Soffer, S. L., Blom-Hoffman, J., & Grim, S. M. (2002). Role of parent training in the effective management of attention-deficit/hyperactivity disorder. *Disease Management and Health Outcomes, 10,* 117–126.

Power, T. J., Shapiro, E. S., & DuPaul, G. J. (in press). Preparing psychologists to link systems of care in managing and preventing health problems: Contributions from school psychology. *Journal of Pediatric Psychology, 27.*

Roberts, M., Carlson, C., Erickson, M., Friedman, R., La Greca, A., Lemanek, K., Russ, S., Schroeder, C., Vargas, L., & Wohlford, P. (1998). A model for training psychologists to provide services for children and adolescents. *Professional Psychology: Research and Practice, 29,* 293–299.

Roberts, M. C. (1998). Innovations in specialty training: The Clinical Child Psychology Program at the University of Kansas. *Professional Psychology: Research and Practice, 29,* 394–397.

Roberts, M. C., & Hurley, L. K. (1997). *Managing managed care.* New York: Plenum Press.

Roberts, M. C., & Steele, R. G. (in press). Predoctoral training in pediatric psychology at the University of Kansas Clinical Child Psychology Program. *Journal of Pediatric Psychology, 27.*

Schwartz, I. S., & Baer, D. M. (1991). Social validity assessments: Is current practice state of the art? *Journal of Applied Behavior Analysis, 24,* 189–204.

Seligman, M. E. P., & Csikszentmihalyi, M. (2000). Positive psychology. *American Psychologist, 55,* 5–14.

Shapiro, E. S., DuPaul, G. J., & Power, T. J. (1997, August). Pediatric school psychology: A new specialty in school health reform. *Pennsylvania Psychologist Quarterly,* pp. 20–21.

Shapiro, E. S., DuPaul, G. J., Power, T. J., Gureasko, S., & Moore, D. (2000, November). Student perspectives on pediatric school psychology. *Communique of the National Association of School Psychologists, 29,* 6–8.

Sheridan, S. M., Kratochwill, T. R., & Bergan, J. R. (1996). *Conjoint behavioral consultation: A procedural manual.* New York: Plenum Press.

Short, R. J., & Talley, R. C. (1997). Rethinking psychology in the schools: Implications of recent national policy. *American Psychologist, 52,* 234–240.

Spirito, A., Brown, R. T., D'Angelo, E., Delameter, A., Rodrique, J., & Siegel, L. (in press). Recommendations for the training of pediatric psychologists. *Journal of Pediatric Psychology, 27,*

Sue, D. W., & Sue, D. (1999). *Counseling the culturally different: Theory and practice* (3rd ed.). New York: Wiley.

Ysseldyke, J., Dawson, P., Lehr, C., Reschly, D., Reynolds, M., & Telzrow, C. (1997). School psychology: A blueprint for training and practice II. Bethesda, MD: National Association of School Psychologists.

CHAPTER 11

Forming Partnerships to Integrate Research and Practice

Research and practice related to the intersection of the family, school, healthcare, and other community-based systems are in an embryonic stage. Our position, as expressed throughout this book, is that the developmental–ecological model provides a road map to guide research and practice related to the health needs of children. The development of the child must be understood in the context of interrelated systems that determine and are determined by the developing child. Just as the child's competencies and needs are constantly evolving, so too are the contexts in which children develop (Sameroff, 1993). The developing child always is contributing to the reconstruction of the interlocking systems that strongly influence his or her development. Furthermore, the ecologies in which the child develops, in turn, exert a strong influence on the direction of the evolving child.

In this final chapter, we provide a brief review of the status of prevention and intervention science with regard to use of a developmental–ecological framework, and we outline some of the challenges in linking research with practice in conducting prevention and intervention studies that integrate systems of care. The chapter concludes with a set of recommendations for conducting prevention and intervention research in a manner that incorporates a developmental–ecological model and facilitates the translation of research into practice.

243

INCORPORATING A DEVELOPMENTAL–ECOLOGICAL FRAMEWORK INTO RESEARCH

Research related to risk–resilience and developmental psychopathology has made significant contributions to our understanding of factors that promote health and competence among children (Masten & Coatsworth, 1998). These factors include characteristics of the child as well as qualities of the contexts in which children develop. This body of research is strongly influencing the direction of prevention science and practice. The thrust of the best prevention work that is being conducted (e.g., Fast Track; Conduct Problems Prevention Research Group, 2002) is to focus on building strong partnerships for children within multiple systems and to integrate systems, so that they work in an orchestrated manner to promote the health of children. Although Fast Track, like many other prevention studies, is an ambitious project that would be highly challenging to replicate in many community settings, this study uses a developmental–ecological framework that accounts for important contexts and relationships that are critical to the developing child.

Unfortunately, the evolution of science and practice related to interventions for health and mental health disorders appears to be progressing at a slower pace than advancements in prevention. Although many leaders in pediatric, clinical, and school psychology are attempting to move intervention science and practice from an exclusive focus on the child to a focus on the interaction of child and context (e.g., Kazak, Simms, & Rourke, 2002; Pianta & Walsh, 1998), very little intervention research has focused on addressing children's needs in multiple contexts and linking systems of care for children (Brown, 2002). Henggeler's work in the area of multisystemic therapy (Henggeler, Melton, & Smith, 1992), Fantuzzo's work related to community partnerships in Head Start (Fantuzzo & Mohr, 2000), and Sheridan's work in conjoint behavioral consultation (Sheridan, Eagle, Cowan, & Mickelson, 2001) are a few of the notable exceptions. It is noteworthy that these exceptions refer to programs addressing the mental health needs of children; there are fewer examples of multisystemic programs that address children's health problems.

Researchers conducting work related to children's healthcare and mental healthcare needs have become increasingly concerned about the translation of research into practice. Although this problem may be related to many factors, including the challenges of conducting research in community-based settings and the failure to prepare professionals to translate research to practice, contingencies established by the National Institutes of Health (NIH) certainly have contributed significantly to this state of affairs (U.S. Department and Health and Human Services, 2001). Historically, the NIH has been much more likely to fund studies related to basic science and research investigating the efficacy of intervention methods under highly controlled conditions. There has been less emphasis on developing and evaluating interventions in community settings and understanding factors that promote the effective dissemination of effective interventions in practice (Dodge, 2001). This tradition appears to be ending. The recently published *Blueprint for Change in Research on Child and Adolescent Mental Health*, developed by the National Institute of Mental Health (NIMH; U.S. Department of Health and Human Services, 2001), outlines an exciting agenda for research and practice in the future. As indicated in this document, NIMH has placed increasing emphasis on the importance of research related to the development of intervention and prevention strategies that are responsive to the needs of professionals working in community settings. Research conducted in an interdisciplinary manner through partnerships formed among scientists at the basic, applied, and community levels is strongly recommended.

CHALLENGES OF TRANSLATING RESEARCH INTO PRACTICE

To understand the challenges at hand, it is useful to consider the four major stages in the development of intervention and prevention methods that are required to link research with practice. These stages include: basic research, efficacy research, effectiveness research, and dissemination research. The stages are outlined in the *Blueprint for Change*, although similar processes have been described by several researchers (e.g., see Dodge, 2001). Table 11.1 provides a brief description of each stage and indicates some of the professional disciplines that typically conduct research within each stage.

Historically, two major problems have precluded movement from one stage to another, particularly in the latter stages. First, as indicated, funding priorities, particularly at the Federal level, typically have favored basic research and intervention efficacy projects. Studies related to evaluating effectiveness and methods of dissemination, typically conducted in community-based settings, generally have not been a priority for Federal funding, although private funding through foundation and corporate grants, and public funding at the state and local levels have supported some projects in these stages. Second, researchers working within each stage typically have conducted their work in isolation from

TABLE 11.1. Stages in the Development of Intervention and Prevention Strategies

Stage	Description	Examples of disciplines
Basic research	Research designed to understand biopsychosocial factors that affect development for the purpose of theory development.	Genetics Neuroradiology Epidemiology Developmental psychology Developmental psychopathology Educational psychology Family psychology Health psychology
Efficacy research	Research designed to investigate the efficacy of an intervention or prevention strategy through controlled clinical trials.	Clinical psychology Pediatric psychology Psychiatry Pediatrics Nursing
Effectiveness research	Research designed to investigate the efficacy, feasibility, and social validity of intervention and prevention strategies in the community.	Community psychology School psychology Public health specialists Community stakeholders
Dissemination research	Research designed to investigate methods for disseminating effective intervention and prevention strategies, and for bringing these methods to full scale.	Public health Public policy specialists Community stakeholders

researchers focusing on other stages. This state of affairs has limited to some extent the utility of basic science and efficacy research for practice, and it has contributed to practice that may be lacking with regard to its theoretical and empirical underpinnings.

To address problems related to the link between science and practice, the NIMH, in the *Blueprint for Change*, has clearly outlined its intention to support research related to each stage of intervention and prevention development. Furthermore, the NIMH has strongly recommended that scientists, community-based professionals, and public health specialists, whose work relates to the continuum from basic to applied work, develop partnerships in conducting their research. The following is a description of some of the challenges of linking the four stages of science in conducting research to address children's health issues within and across multiple systems of care.

Linking Basic and Applied Science:
Developing a Foundation for Practice

Basic science investigating biopsychosocial factors that contribute to development within multiple systems of care involves a wide range of specialties. At the level of the individual child, scientists conducting research in the fields of genetics, neuroradiology, neuropharmacology, epidemiology, developmental neuropsychiatry and neuropsychology, and developmental psychology, among others, are making highly important contributions that can have an impact on intervention development. At the level of systems, research related to family psychology and developmental psychopathology is advancing our understanding of family factors that promote health and contribute to reduction of health risk among children and adolescents. Basic research in educational psychology and organizational development has contributed greatly to our understanding of school ecology and factors that promote cognitive and social development, and family involvement in school. Nursing and public health, among other disciplines, are advancing our understanding of systems of healthcare and variables related to access and quality of care. Social psychology and sociology have contributed greatly to our understanding of formal and informal institutions in the community that address the healthcare and developmental needs of children.

Conducting basic research that has the potential to be clinically relevant requires collaborations among professionals at the basic and applied levels. These partnerships may involve professionals from multiple disciplines and often several divisions within the same discipline (U.S. Department of Health and Human Services, 2001). Through collaboration, basic researchers can be held accountable to investigate issues that have the potential to contribute to intervention development. Simultaneously, these partnerships offer applied researchers a framework for developing interventions that are grounded in well-substantiated theories, and therefore have the potential to be successful and contribute to the further development of theory.

Applied scientists, in their efforts to design intervention and prevention strategies to address the health concerns of children, need to understand development in the context of the systems that have an impact on health (Brown, 2002; Pianta, 2001). For example, researchers devising psychosocial interventions for children and families coping with cancer need to incorporate an understanding of the disease, principles of child development, family research related to coping with disease, and evidence-based family and cognitive-behavioral intervention strategies to design potentially efficacious interventions (see Kazak et al., 1999). Likewise, researchers developing psychosocial interventions for children with ADHD in family and school settings need to understand the disorder and its developmental course, family research related to parent–child relationships, educational research related to teacher consultation and family–school collaboration, and evidence-based strategies of practice (see Power, Karustis, & Habboushe, 2001). Through collaborations with basic scientists conducting research within multiple systems of care, applied researchers can develop intervention programs that are comprehensive and scientifically grounded.

Linking Efficacy and Effectiveness Research: Translating Research to Practice

Efficacy studies, or clinical trials, attempt to investigate the outcomes of interventions under highly controlled conditions. Typically the intervention being investigated is compared with one or more control groups to determine its relative efficacy. The interventionists in these studies often are highly trained and well-supervised graduate students or research assistants. Interventionists are trained to a well-specified criterion level, and the integrity with which they apply procedures is monitored extremely carefully. The strengths of this research include the incorporation of intervention strategies with at least preliminary empirical support, commitment to a high standard of practice, and use of multimethod outcome evaluation procedures.

Efficacy studies have noteworthy limitations, however. One concern is that efficacy studies are conducted in a manner that may be very different from that in community-based practice. Although research assistants involved in efficacy studies may be meticulous in implementing intervention strategies, they may do so in a way that lacks responsiveness to the cultural values and developmental needs of children and their families. Furthermore, efficacy studies may not take into account the real-life feasibility issues that can have an impact on service delivery in the community (e.g., restrictions imposed by managed care, variable level of training and expertise among professional staff, and overwhelming referral rates and waiting lists).

Effectiveness refers to multiple domains of outcome, in addition to efficacy. Effective interventions are those that are feasible for practitioners to implement given the contingencies and parameters existing in community-based practice. Moreover, effective treatments, by definition, are socially valid to the major stakeholders. Social validity refers to the extent to which the goals, methods, and intended outcomes of intervention are perceived by stakeholders as reasonable, appropriate, and fair (Kazdin, 1981; Schwartz & Baer, 1991). Socially valid methods are responsive to the cultural values and priorities of families, and developmentally appropriate for the children being served. To the extent that intervention and prevention methods are feasible and socially valid, practitioners and families generally are willing to sustain their use throughout the period of intervention and follow-up (Witt & Elliott, 1985).

Linking efficacy and effectiveness research involves applying evidence-based practices supported through efficacy research in a manner that is feasible and socially valid in community-based practice, which may involve practitioners from a wide range of disciplines, as well as paraprofessionals in roles as intervention providers (see Dowrick et al., 2001). Doing so requires close collaboration between researchers, practitioners, and paraprofessionals. Partnership-based or participatory action research methods are highly useful in developing intervention and prevention strategies that can inform community-based practice and be viewed by providers and clients as appropriate and potentially useful (see Israel, Schulz, Parker, & Becker, 1998). These methods applied to research addressing the health issues of children across systems mandate the active participation of many constituents, including researchers, community-based providers from the school and healthcare systems, caregivers, and children themselves (Connell, Kubisch, Schorr, & Weiss, 1995). In a partnership framework, these stakeholders are engaged in a nonhierarchical, co-construction process from the outset through every stage of intervention development and outcome evaluation (Fantuzzo, Coolahan, & Weiss, 1997; Nastasi et al., 2000).

Bringing Interventions to Scale: Addressing the Challenges of Dissemination

Even when interventions have been co-constructed by researchers, providers, and families, and validated for use in community settings, disseminating this information to practitioners and facilitating widescale use of interventions can be highly challenging. Very little research has been conducted regarding barriers to transportability and strategies to overcome these obstacles. Quite simply, what is needed are evidence-based practices for disseminating evidence-based intervention and prevention practices into diverse communities (U.S. Department of Health and Human Services, 2001).

A common misconception is that interventions developed and validated for use in one community can be implemented with little or no adaptation in another community (Elias & Branden, 1988). Dissemination strategies involving information distribution, although useful, are limited in their effectiveness. Critical elements of intervention dissemination may be very similar to those for intervention development and evaluation. Transportability requires effective, ongoing collaboration between trainers and practitioners, as well as their clients. Trainers seeking to transport evidence-based practices into diverse settings need to form partnerships with stakeholders in these communities. Through these partnerships, trainers and community stakeholders can negotiate ways of adapting evidence-based practices in a manner that is developmentally appropriate and culturally responsive for children and families residing in the community (Dowrick et al., 2001).

Bringing intervention and prevention programs to scale requires the intersection of the research community with the public policy sector. Historically, intervention and prevention researchers have conducted their work with little regard for public policy issues. Programs have been developed without a consideration of the challenges in full-scale implementation (Dodge, 2001). Forming partnerships with policymakers from the outset and collaborating with these officials throughout the process of research can enable investigators to conduct research in a manner that has the potential to shape public policy.

RECOMMENDATIONS FOR THE FUTURE

Given these challenges, what steps can be taken in the near future to link research with practice in a way that will promote the healthy development of children across the multiple systems in which they operate? The short answer is to *form partnerships*. The following are some specific ideas about the kinds of partnerships that researchers and practitioners can develop to create healthy systems for children and to facilitate linkages among systems of care.

Create Partnerships among Basic, Clinical, Community, and Public Health Researchers

As indicated, the tradition is for researchers at each level of science (i.e., basic, clinical, community, and public healthcare) to collaborate with other investigators within the same level. These partnerships are limited and do not address the challenges outlined in the previous section. Multidisciplinary partnerships among researchers at every level of investigation are needed to link the stages of research and to facilitate the implementation of theoretically and empirically grounded intervention and prevention strategies in community-based practice (U.S. Department of Health and Human Services, 2001). What this means is that developmental psychologists and experts in developmental psychopathology need to collaborate with psychiatrists and clinical/pediatric psychologists in developing prevention and intervention strategies. Clinical/pediatric psychologists and psychiatrists should collaborate with community, school, and family psychologists, as well as public health experts to develop potentially effective community-based treatments. Clinical and community researchers need to work in partnership with public health professionals and policy experts to translate research findings into policies that can make a difference for large groups of children.

Form Partnerships among Professionals Using Varying Paradigms and Methodologies

Health-related professionals often differ greatly in the paradigms that form the basis of their professional activities and in the methodologies they use to address research and programmatic challenges. These variations often are rooted in fundamental differences in training programs across disciplines, as well as across divisions within the same discipline. For example, training in psychiatry typically is based on the medical model, which may be reflected in the predominance of categorical methods of assessment. In contrast, training in psychology often is reactive to the medical model and typically advances a multidimensional framework that espouses that emotional and behavioral functioning vary along a continuum, from highly adaptive to highly maladaptive. However, psychology itself consists of highly divergent paradigms with contrasting methodologies. For example, behavior analysts employ methodologies based on the experimental analysis of behavior; developmental–ecological psychologists emphasize methods for understanding and improving adult and peer relationships; and cognitive-behavioral psychologists emphasize the use of methods to understand and change the thinking patterns of individuals and the relationship of these patterns to behavior.

The paradigms that form the basis of varying approaches to research and practice are each based on a unique set of assumptions. In general, each paradigm is associated with numerous strengths, as well as limitations. Unfortunately, professionals practicing within each of these traditions often fail to recognize the limitations of the paradigms from which they operate, and they also may fail to acknowledge the strengths of alternative paradigms. Over time, professionals who establish their work on a particular theoretical basis may become isolated from those who ground their activities in other paradigms (Sternberg & Grigorenko, 2001). As a result, research and practice that operates within a particular tradition are limited by the shortcomings of the paradigm and are deprived from benefiting from the assets of alternative, at times complementary, paradigms.

To address this problem, it is essential that researchers and practitioners who base their work on divergent paradigms form partnerships with each other (Sternberg & Grigorenko, 2001). Through these collaborations, professionals can develop multiple perspectives for understanding issues and create methods of inquiry and validation that integrate several different methodologies.

Develop Partnerships among Professionals across Systems of Care

Historically, researchers and practitioners have collaborated with professionals who work within the same system (La Greca & Hughes, 1999). For example, pediatric psychologists typically collaborate with physicians and other health professionals in conducting their work; clinical psychologists generally limit their collaborations to professionals in the mental health system; and school psychologists collaborate primarily with educational professionals. This arrangement fails to promote the integration of systems and fails to incorporate professionals with diverse perspectives in the development of intervention and prevention programs that address children's functioning across systems. So what is needed are partnerships among pediatric and school professionals to develop interventions that facilitate children's functioning in the family, school, and healthcare system, and that promote partnerships among these systems (Power, Shapiro, & DuPaul, in press). Likewise, partnerships between primary care pediatric providers and pediatric psychologists can improve the medical management of children with common health problems and address the mental health needs of these children (Brown & Freeman, 2002; Drotar, 1995).

Establish Partnerships with Diverse Stakeholder Groups

Intervention and prevention programs have an impact on stakeholder groups from multiple systems. Unfortunately, programs typically involve representatives from a limited number of stakeholder groups. Not surprisingly, researchers and practitioner groups may be disproportionately represented, and stakeholders from diverse community systems (e.g., schools, mental healthcare system, and other formal and informal community organizations), as well as public policy officials, often are underrepresented. Successful research, that is, research that has the potential to have an impact on practice and can make a difference in the lives of children and families, involves representatives from each major stakeholder group throughout all stages of the program (Connell et al., 1995). Participatory action research methods are highly useful in building partnerships to design, implement, and evaluate programs that are meaningful to diverse stakeholders and have the potential to have an impact at multiples levels (see Nastasi et al., 2000).

CONCLUSIONS

Addressing children's health issues from both an intervention and a prevention standpoint involves working within and across multiple systems. Psychology is at an early stage in developing models to manage and prevent children's health problems across systems, although developmental–ecological theory provides a framework to guide research and practice for the foreseeable future.

Numerous barriers have impeded progress in conducting research and translating research to practice related to the management and prevention of health problems across systems. One problem has been that the research community is fractionated. Researchers operating at the basic level often conduct their work in isolation from applied researchers who are developing innovative strategies to address children's health issues. This results in basic science that is lacking in clinical utility and clinical practice with insufficient theoretical and empirical grounding. Another problem is that applied researchers and community-based practitioners work in isolation from each other, thereby resulting in a failure of practice concerns to shape research, and a failure of research to inform practice. A further concern is that the research community and policy sector often operate in different spheres and fail to work in collaboration, resulting in effective practices that are disseminated poorly, and public policy that is not consistent with evidence-based practice.

A major challenge to the research, practice, and policy sectors is to form meaningful partnerships with one another at the outset of intervention/prevention development and throughout every stage of the process. To address children's health issues, this process requires the involvement of stakeholders at the academic, practice, and policy levels representing multiple systems, including the family, school, healthcare and mental healthcare systems, and other formal and informal organizations in the community. Models of research developed by anthropologists and community psychologists (e.g., participatory research, action research, partnership-based research) have the potential to guide the process of forming partnerships across the research, practice, and public policy sectors to conduct highly meaningful research with the potential for social change. Standards for determining the quality of research must not only continue to emphasize the need for a high level of methodological rigor but should also reflect the potential for research to contribute to effective practice and to shape policy. Finally, training programs need to place a priority on enabling future professionals to form meaningful partnerships across levels of research, systems of healthcare, and paradigms for promoting change.

REFERENCES

Brown, R. T. (2002). Society of pediatric psychology presidential address: Toward a social ecology of pediatric psychology. *Journal of Pediatric Psychology, 27,* 191–202.

Brown, R. T., & Freeman, W. (2002). Primary care. In L. Marsh & M. Fristad (Eds.), *Handbook of serious emotional disturbance in children and adolescents* (pp. 428–444). New York: Wiley.

Conduct Problems Prevention Research Group. (2002). The implementation of the Fast Track program: An example of a large-scale prevention science efficacy trial. *Journal of Abnormal Child Psychology, 30,* 1–18.

Connell, J. P., Kubisch, A. C., Schorr, L. B., & Weiss, C. H. (Eds.), (1995). *New approaches to evaluating community initiatives: Concepts, methods, and contexts.* Washington, DC: Aspen Institute.

Dodge, K. A. (2001). The science of youth violence prevention: Progressing from developmental epidemiology to efficacy to effectiveness to public policy. *American Journal of Preventive Medicine, 20 (1S),* 63–70.

Dowrick, P. W., Power, T. J., Manz, P. H., Ginsburg-Block, M., Leff, Stephen, S., & Kim-Rupnow, S. (2001). Community responsiveness: Examples from under-resourced urban schools. *Journal of Prevention and Intervention in the Community, 21,* 71–90.

Drotar, D. (1995). *Consulting with pediatricians: Psychological perspectives for research and practice.* New York: Plenum Press.

Elias, M. J., & Branden, L. R. (1988). Primary prevention of behavioral and emotional problems in school-aged populations. *School Psychology Review, 17,* 581–592.

Fantuzzo, J. W., Coolahan, K., & Weiss, A. (1997). Resiliency partnership-directed research: Enhancing the social competencies of preschool victims of physical abuse by developing peer resources and community strengths. In D. Cicchetti & S. Toth (Eds.), *Developmental perspective on trauma: Theory, research and intervention* (pp. 463–514). Rochester, NY: University of Rochester Press.

Fantuzzo, J. W., & Mohr, W. (2000). Pursuit of wellness in Head Start: Making beneficial connections for children and families. In D. Cicchetti, J. Rapapport, I. Sandler, & R. Weissberg (Eds.), *The promotion of wellness in children and adolescents* (pp. 463–514). Thousand Oaks, CA: Sage.

Henggeler, S. W., Melton, G. B., & Smith, L. A. (1992). Family preservation using multisystemic therapy: An effective alternative to incarcerating serious juvenile offenders. *Journal of Consulting and Clinical Psychology, 60,* 953–961.

Israel, B. A., Schulz, A. J., Parker, E. A., & Becker, A. B. (1998). Review of community-based research: Assessing partnership approaches to improve public health. *Annual Review of Public Health, 19,* 173–202.

Kazak, A. E., Simms, S., Barakat, L., Hobbie, W., Foley, B., Golomb, V., & Best, M. (1999). Surviving cancer competently intervention program (SCCIP): A cognitive-behavioral and family therapy intervention for adolescent survivors of childhood cancer and their families. *Family Process, 38,* 175–191.

Kazak, A. E., Simms, S., & Rourke, M. T. (2002). Family systems practice in pediatric psychology. *Journal of Pediatric Psychology, 27,* 133–145.

Kazdin, A. E. (1981). Acceptability of child treatment techniques: The influence of treatment efficacy and adverse side effects. *Behavior Therapy, 12,* 493–506.

La Greca, A. M., & Hughes, J. N. (1999). United we stand, divided we fall: The education and training of clinical child psychologists. *Journal of Clinical Child Psychology, 28,* 435–447.

Masten, A. S., & Coatsworth, J. D. (1998). The development of competence in favorable and unfavorable environments: Lessons from research on successful children. *American Psychologist, 53,* 205–220.

Nastasi, B. K., Varjas, K., Schensul, S. L., Silva, K. T., Schensul, J. J., & Ratnayake, P. (2000). The participatory intervention model: A framework for conceptualizing and promoting intervention acceptability. *School Psychology Quarterly, 15,* 207–232.

Pianta, R. C. (2001). Implications of a developmental systems model for preventing and treating behavioral disturbances in children and adolescents. In J. N. Hughes, A. M. La Greca, & J. C. Conoley (Eds.), *Handbook of psychological services for children and adolescents* (pp. 23–42). New York: Oxford University Press.

Pianta, R. C., & Walsh, D. J. (1998). Applying the construct of resilience in schools: Cautions from a developmental systems perspective. *School Psychology Review, 27,* 407–417.

Power, T. J., Karustis, J. L., & Habboushe, D. F. (2001). *Homework success for children with ADHD: A family–school intervention program.* New York: Guilford Press.

Power, T. J., Shapiro, E. S., & DuPaul, G. J. (in press). Preparing psychologists to link the health and educational systems in managing and preventing children's health problems. *Journal of Pediatric Psychology.*

Sameroff, A. J. (1993). Models of development and developmental risk. In C. H. Zeanah (Ed.), *Handbook of infant mental health* (pp. 3–13). New York: Guilford Press.

Schwartz, I. S., & Baer, D. M. (1991). Social validity assessments: Is current practice state of the art? *Journal of Applied Behavior Analysis, 24,* 189–204.

Sheridan, S. M., Eagle, J. W., Cowan, R. J., & Mickelson, W. (2001). The effects of conjoint behavioral consultation: Results of a 4-year investigation. *Journal of School Psychology, 39,* 361–385.

Sternberg, R. J., & Grigorenko, E. L. (2001). Unified psychology. *American Psychologist, 56,* 1069–1079.

U.S. Department of Health and Human Services. (2001). *Blueprint for change:*

Research on child and adolescent mental health. Washington, DC: Department of Health and Human Services, Public Health Service, National Institutes of Health, National Institute of Mental Health.

Witt, J. C., & Elliott, S. N. (1985). Acceptability of classroom intervention strategies. In T. R. Kratochwill (Ed.), *Advances in school psychology* (Vol. 4, pp. 251–288). Hillsdale, NJ: Erlbaum.

Index

f refers to a figure; *t* refers to a table